Lifeboat Design and Development No.8

WAVE[NEY]

FAST AFLOAT LIFEBOATS

The RNLI's Waveney class lifeboats, their design and history

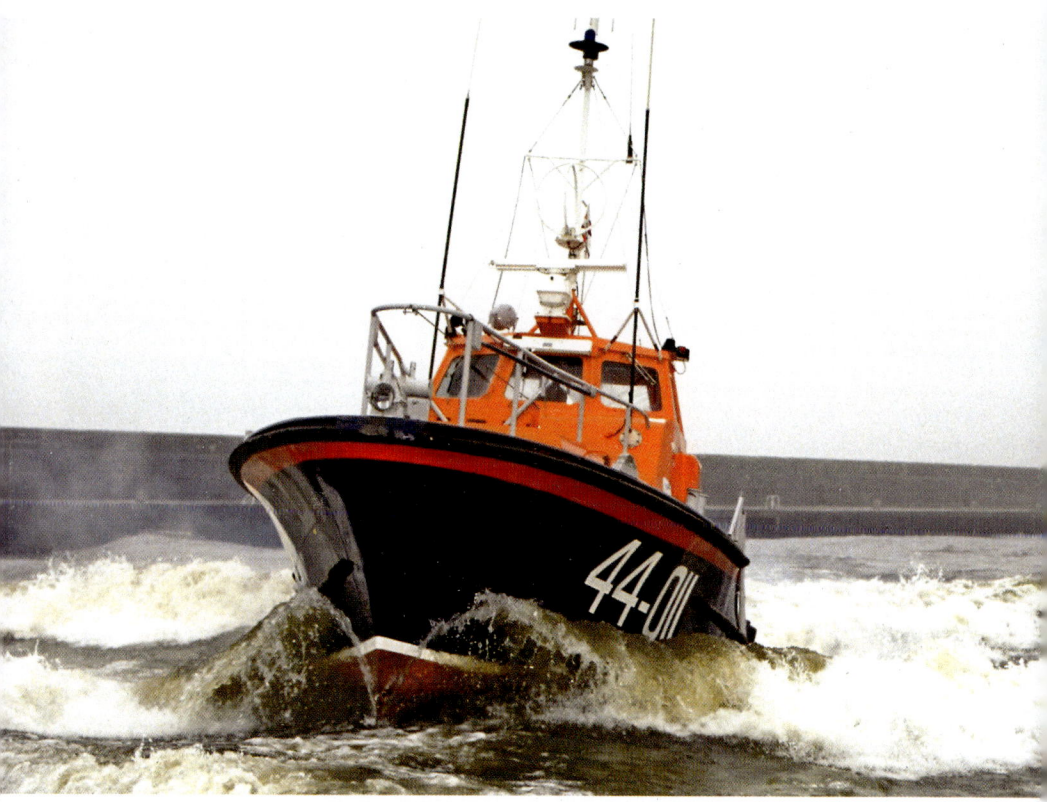

Nicholas Leach

FOXGLOVE PUBLISHING

First published 2022

Published by
Foxglove Publishing Ltd
Foxglove House, Shute Hill,
Lichfield WS13 8DB
United Kingdom
Tel 07940 905046

ISBN 9781909540231

Typesetting/layout by
Nicholas Leach/
Foxglove Publishing

LIFEBOAT BOOKS PUBLISHED BY FOXGLOVE PUBLISHING

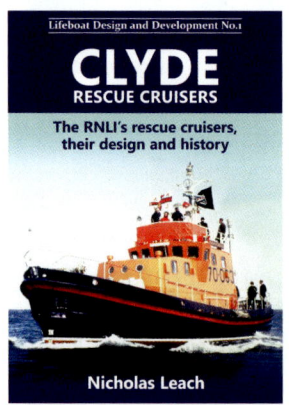

Lifeboat Design and Development No.1

CLYDE
RESCUE CRUISERS

The RNLI's rescue cruisers,
their design and history

Nicholas Leach

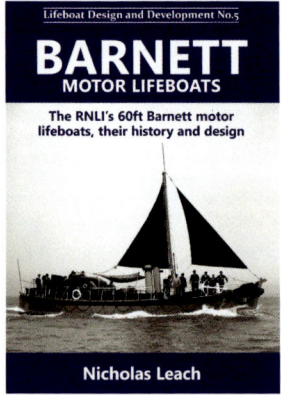

Lifeboat Design and Development No.5

BARNETT
MOTOR LIFEBOATS

The RNLI's 60ft Barnett motor
lifeboats, their history and design

Nicholas Leach

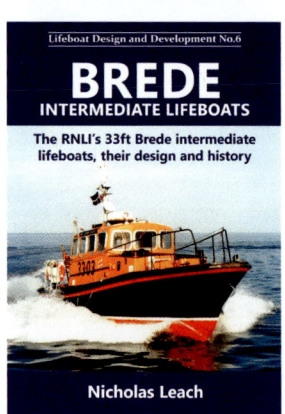

Lifeboat Design and Development No.6

BREDE
INTERMEDIATE LIFEBOATS

The RNLI's 33ft Brede intermediate
lifeboats, their design and history

Nicholas Leach

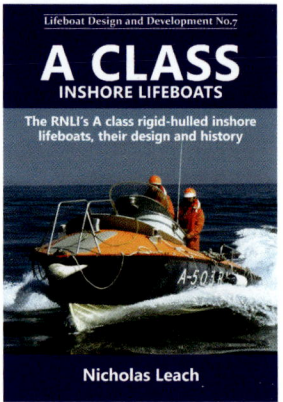

Lifeboat Design and Development No.7

A CLASS
INSHORE LIFEBOATS

The RNLI's A class rigid-hulled inshore
lifeboats, their design and history

Nicholas Leach

LIFEBOAT DESIGN AND DEVELOPMENT SERIES This is the eighth book in a series of concise illustrated volumes that trace the history of and describe technical aspects of RNLI motor lifeboat types. The first volume in the series covered the Clyde class rescue cruisers, the RNLI's largest lifeboats; the second detailed the Surf motor lifeboats; the third covered the Atlantic rigid-inflatable inshore lifeboats; the fourth looked at the 47ft Tyne fast slipway lifeboats, the last of which left active service in 2019; .

THE AUTHOR Nicholas Leach has a long-standing interest in lifeboats and the lifeboat service. He has written many articles, books and papers on the subject, including a history of the origins of the lifeboat service; a comprehensive record of the RNLI's lifeboat stations in 1999, the organisation's 175th anniversary; RNLI Motor Lifeboats, a detailed history of the development of powered lifeboats; and numerous station histories, including ones covering the stations of Cromer, Longhope, Padstow, Sennen Cove, Weymouth and Humber. He has visited all of the lifeboat stations in the UK and Ireland, past and present, and is Editor of Ships Monthly, the international shipping magazine, and Lifeboats Past & Present, the magazine for lifeboat enthusiasts.

Contents

Acknowledgements

Many people have assisted with this publication, and I am grateful to them all. Hayley Whiting of the RNLI Heritage Trust has made research facilities available at the RNLI over many years. Ian Moignard thoroughly checked the text and the facts, and I am extremely grateful to him. Clive Lawford kindly assisted with finding various images of Waveneys as they are in the 2020s, and his website dedicated to the 44ft lifeboats (www.44mlb.com) is a goldmine of information and is highly recommended. My thanks to the various people also supplied photographs for possible inclusion: Martin Fish, David Forshaw, Cliff Crone, Peter Edey, Gary Markham, Hilmar Snorrason, William D. Wilkinson and Victor Young. I have made every effort to correctly credit the photographs, but this has not been possible with every image, and my apologies to those whose names are not recorded.

Nicholas Leach, Lichfield, March 2022

Summary of the RNLI's 44ft Waveney lifeboats

Op No	ON	Year	Name	Cost	Engines (twin diesels)
44-001	—	1964	[Un-named]	—	2x200hp Cummins V6 1973– 2x250hp Ford Mermaid 595T 1982- 2x203hp Caterpillar 3208
44-002	1001	1966	John F. Kennedy	£38,749	2x215hp Cummins V6 1983– 2x203hp Caterpillar D3208
44-003	1002	1967	Khami	£38,112	2x215hp Cummins V6 1981– 2x203hp Caterpillar D3208
44-004	1003	1967	Faithful Forester	£37,985	2x215hp Cummins V6 1982– 2x203hp Caterpillar D3208
44-005	1004	1967	Margaret Graham	£43,020	2x215hp Cummins V6 1982– 2x203hp Caterpillar D3208
44-006	1005	1968	Arthur and Blanche Harris	£38,318	2x215hp Cummins V6 1979– 2x203hp Caterpillar D3208
44-007	1006	1968	Connel Elizabeth Cargill	£38,343	2x215hp Cummins V6 1982– 2x203hp Caterpillar D3208
44-008	1026	1974	Eric Seal (Civil Service No.36)	£81,864	2x260hp General Motors GM 8V-53
44-009	1027	1974	Helen Turnbull	£73,271	2x260hp General Motors GM 8V-53
44-010	1028	1974	Thomas Forehead and Mary Rowse II	£68,736	2x260hp General Motors GM 8V-53
44-011	1029	1974	Augustine Courtauld	£68.736	2x260hp General Motors GM 8V-53
44-012	1033	1974	White Rose of Yorkshire	£79,018	2x260hp General Motors GM 8V-53
44-013	1034	1974	Thomas James King	£79,049	2x260hp General Motors GM 8V-53
44-014	1035	1974	St Patrick	£79,582	2x260hp General Motors GM 8V-53
44-015	1036	1975	Lady of Lancashire	£85,967	2x260hp General Motors GM 8V-53
44-016	1042	1976	Ralph and Joy Swann	£128,525	2x250hp Ford Mermaid 595T 1981– 2x250hp Caterpillar D3208T
44-017	1043	1976	The Nelsons of Donaghadee/ Wavy Line	£174,688	2x250hp Ford Mermaid 595T 1978– 2x250hp Caterpillar D3208T 1980– 2x250hp Caterpillar D3208T
44-018	1044	1977	The Scout	£129,080	2x250hp Ford Mermaid 595T 1982– 2x250hp Caterpillar D3208T
44-019	1045	1977	Louis Marchesi of Round Table	£139,823	2x250hp Ford Mermaid 595T 1981– 2x250hp Caterpillar D3208T
44-020	1060	1980	John Fison	£243,487	2x250hp Caterpillar 3208T
44-021	1065	1980	Barham	£264,914	2x250hp Caterpillar 3208T
44-022	1079	1982	The William and Jane	£319,940	2x250hp Caterpillar D3208T

Introduction

In July 1999 the last of the 44ft Waveney class lifeboats was taken out of service by the Royal National Lifeboat Institution (RNLI). For more than a quarter of a century, Waveney lifeboats had been stationed throughout the United Kingdom and Ireland, and the well-liked boats had given outstanding service, performing many outstanding rescues in the course of their duties. This book is a tribute to Waveney, an outstanding and ground-breaking design, being the first British lifeboat type to be capable of speeds greater than nine knots.

The 44ft motor lifeboat was designed, developed and built in the United States in the early 1960s. The 44-footer, as it was known, was built for the United States Coast Guard and ws intended primarily to carry out search and rescue work under heavy sea and surf conditions. Such was the outstanding nature of the design, that variants were used around the world, and 44ft motor lifeboats gave service not only in

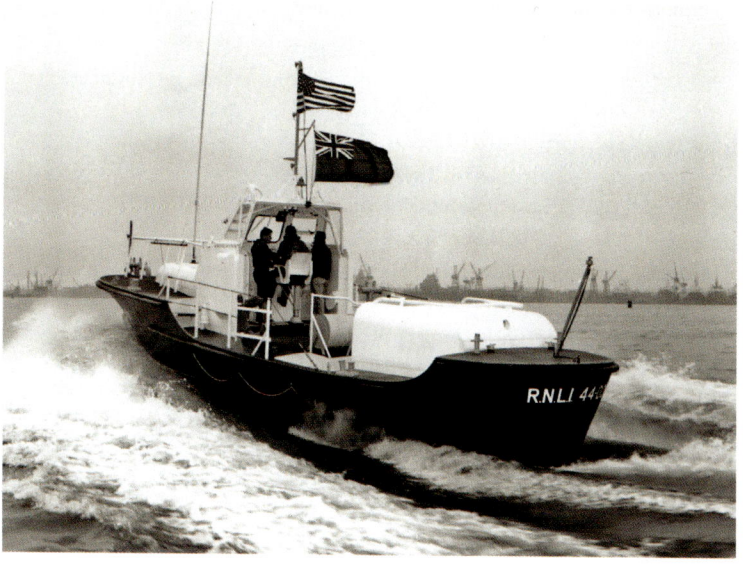

◀ RNLI prototype 44-001, the first Waveney, during her initial trials in America, where she was built. Seen from the port quarter, 44-001 has both US and British ensigns hoisted, symbolising the close cooperation between the two countries to develop improved lifeboat types. (Official USCG photo, from the collection of William Wilkinson)

the United States but also in the United Kingdom and Ireland, and in Canada, Portugal, Norway and Italy, as well as Iran.

This book focusses on the design as used by the Royal National Lifeboat Institution in the United Kingdom and Ireland, where it was designated the Waveney class lifeboat. The design was the first fast lifeboat to see service in British waters, that is a lifeboat capable of more than nine knots, and as such represents the beginning of the modern era of lifeboat design. The worldwide influence on lifeboat development of the 44ft motor lifeboat is testament to its outstanding design and build quality, which encompassed seaworthiness, ease of handling, good speed, and strength and durability that was second to none, as well as excellent towin capabilities. It represents aguably the most significant advance in lifeboat design of the twenieth century.

Bibliography

Dutton, Lieut Commdr W L G (1967): The Development of the 44ft USCG Steel Lifeboat, in Item No.3 in Report on the Tenth International Lifeboat Conference held in Dinard 1967, pp.23-25.

Fry, Eric (1975): Lifeboat Design and Development (David & Charles, London).

Leach, Nicholas (2001): The Waveney Lifeboats: An illustrated history of the RNLI 44ft Waveney lifeboats 1967-1999 (Bernard McCall, Portishead, Bristol).

MacDonald, S., et al (1975): RNLI Lifeboats in the 1970s, Royal Institute of Naval Architects, pp.301-324.

Morris, Jeff (1986): Lists of British Life-boats, Part III: Motor Lifeboats.

Noble, Dennis (2000): Lifeboat Sailors: Disasters, Rescues and the perilous future of the Coast Guard's Small Boat Stations (Brassey's, Washington DC).

Smith, Richard R. (1963): Operational Characteristics of the United States Coast Guard 44-foot Motor Lifeboat, Item No.6 in Report on the Ninth International Lifeboat Conference held in Edinburgh, June 1963, pp.66-70.

Wilkinson, William D (1998): The US Coast Guard 44-foot Motor Lifeboat, in Quarterdeck, newsletter for Columbia River Maritime Museum, Vol.24, No.1, Winter 1998.

Witter, Robert W, Lt Cdr (1963): Design and Construction of the United States Coast Guard 44-foot Motor Lifeboat, Item No.5 in Report on the Ninth International Lifeboat Conference held in Edinburgh, June 1963, pp.51-65.

T he 44ft motor lifeboat has its origins in the rescue work of the United States Coast Guard and its motor lifeboat programme. The first motor lifeboat to see service in the USA, a standard 34ft self-righting lifeboat retro-fitted with a 12hp petrol engine, was trialled by the United States Life-saving Service (USLSS) in 1899. The success of this boat led to many other 34ft lifeboats having engines installed. Improvements in engine technology continued and, in 1907, the first lifeboat designed from the keel up as a motor lifeboat entered service.

The US Coast Guard was formed during the First World War, coming into existence in 1915 when the USLSS was merged with the US Revenue

▼ The standard 36ft USCG Type T lifeboat, seen here with an open aft cockpit, had a speed of about eight knots. (USCG photo)

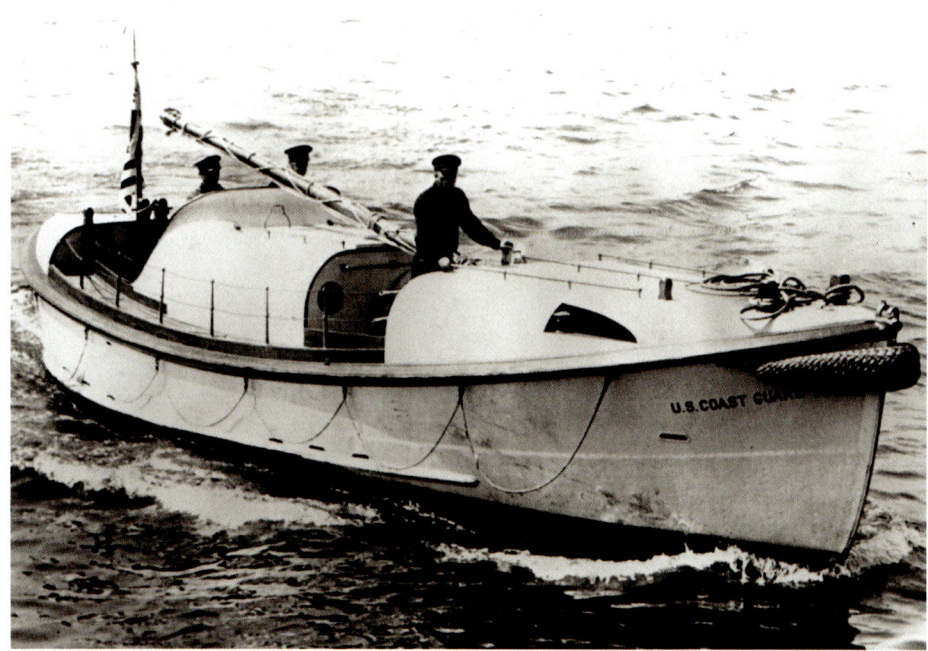

Cutter Service, with the new service becoming fully responsible for search and rescue round America's coasts. Although law enforcement operations were also part of the organisation's remit, a large network of lifeboat stations, known as 'units', was maintained for rescue work, and the newly-created United States Coast Guard continued the work started by USLSS of developing improved motor lifeboat designs.

The first new USCG motor lifeboat, the Type H, was introduced in 1918, its initial development having been slowed when the USA entered the war in 1917. The first Type H was completed by the Curtis Bay Yard in March 1919, and had its propeller enclosed by a semi-tunnel. The next new design was the Type T, which was developed in 1928, and was later modified to the Type TR and Type TRS. This 36ft 8in self-bailing and self-righting single-engined craft became the mainstay of the USCG lifeboat fleet until production ceased in 1956, but the boats remained in service for many years after.

The 36-footers, as they were known, were fitted with a single 90hp petrol engine which gave a speed of about eight knots and a cruising radius of almost 200 miles. Most were kept afloat, although some were carriage launched and kept in a boathouse. USCG personnel reached

▼ The USCG's Type TR motor lifeboat CG36363 from Station Short Beach, New York. The Type TR was a very successful design, and remained largely unchanged throughout the build programme. (USCG photo)

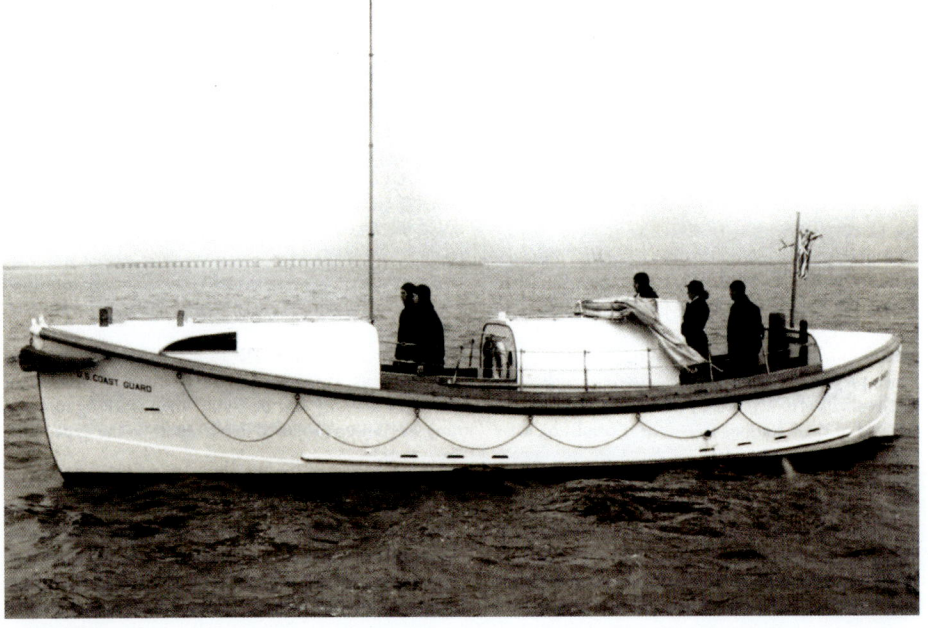

WAVENEY LIFEBOATS

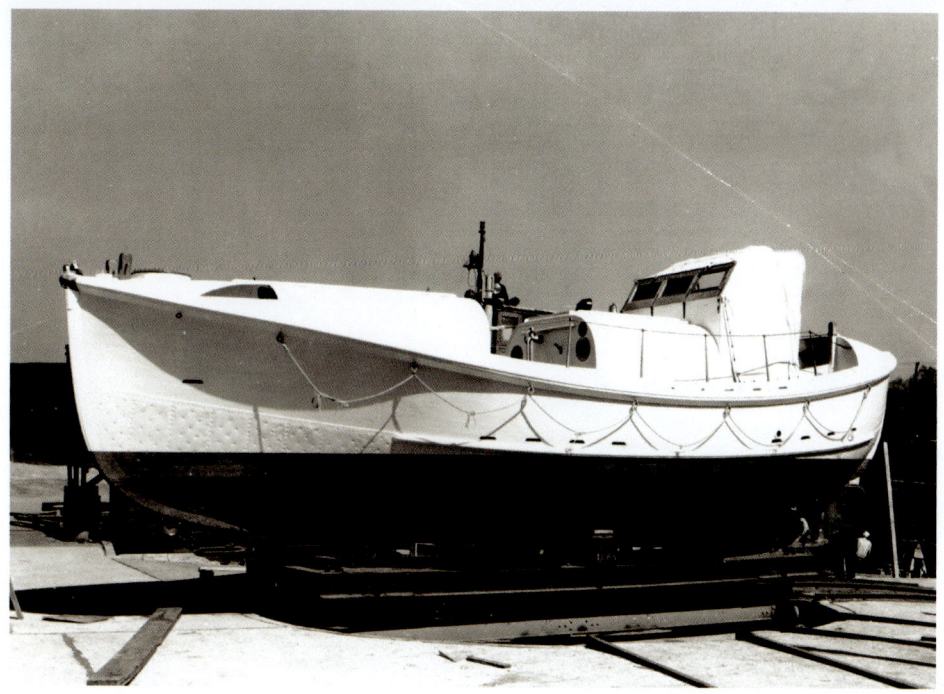

a high degree of proficiency in handling this lifeboat, which proved its worth in many rescues both at the coast and on the Great Lakes, and was the workhorse of the service for many years. However, by the 1960s, a decade which began with 150 boats of this type in service, the design was beginning to show its age. The boats themselves had an average age of nineteen years, and, not only were they showing definite signs of wear, but they were no longer meeting the operational requirements of the USCG. Recreational boating in the United States had increased considerably during the 1950s, and the country's coastal waters had become densely populated with a variety of small craft.

▲ A newly completed 36-footer ready for shipment to the coast; the design had a displacement hull, with the aft cockpit partially enclosed. (USCG photo)

When the weather worsened, recreational boaters and small commercial fishermen were getting into trouble. As speed was crucial in reaching these casualties, a 40ft utility boat, capable of twenty-one knots, entered service to supplement the 36-footer and provide routine assistance in fair weather. In rough weather, however, the 36-footer was called upon. Consequently many stations had to operate two vessels, an unnecessary expense, particularly when one of these boats, the slow 36-footer, was poorly suited to the high volume of work it had to

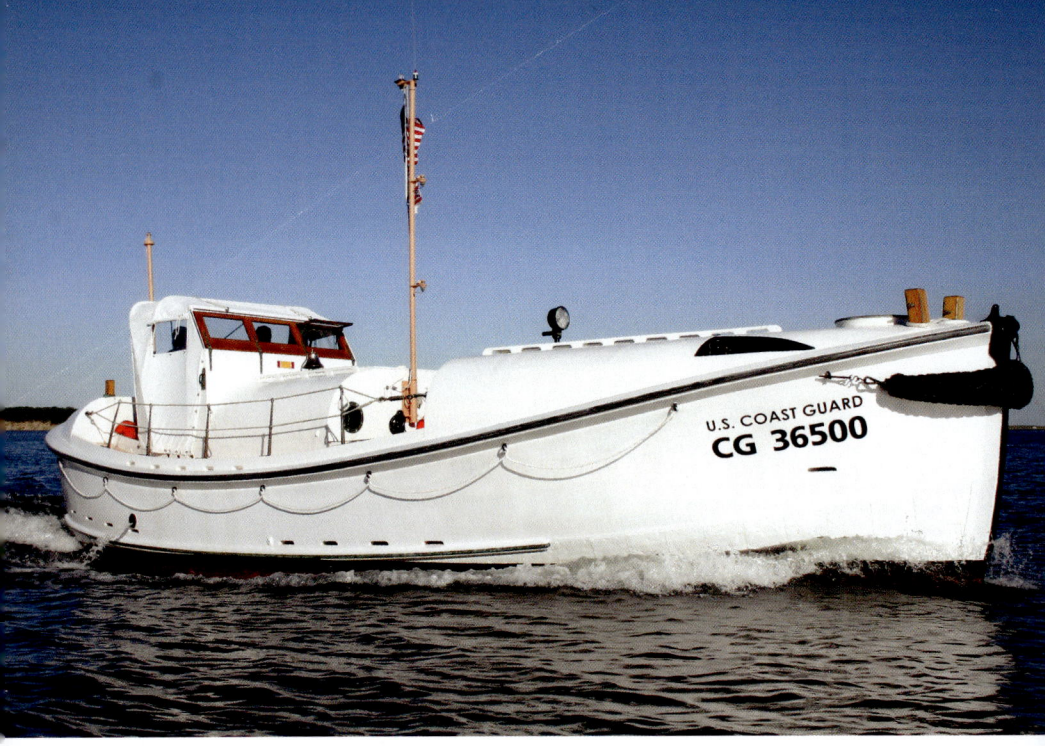

▲ CG-36500 was built in 1946 at the Coast Guard Yard in Curtis Bay, Baltimore, where all 36-footers were built. Typical of the type which was replaced by the 44-footer, CG-36500 is notable for her involvement in the rescue in 1952 of the steamer Pendleton, one of the most daring such events in the history of the USCG. (Nicholas Leach)

undertake. What was needed was a new design of faster, all-weather craft, which could perform the roles of both the 40ft and the 36ft craft.

In developing a new design, the main operational shortcomings of the 36-footers were identified. These were poor towing control due to the far aft location of the towing bollard, lack of speed, and poor visibility from the steering position. However, the design had its strengths and the crews who operated the boats stressed these must be kept. In designing a new boat, seaworthiness, self-righting capability and compartmentation, all integral to the 36-footer, could not be compromised. The new design had to be both fast and able to operate in the worst of weathers. It also had to have all relevant electronic equipment, including radar, direction finder, echo sounder and radio. In addition, it had to have twin screws, a range of 150 nautical miles at full speed, provision for survivors, engine-driven fire and salvage pump, excellent towing capability and an integrated steering and control console.

Development of the 44ft motor lifeboat

Once the requirements of the new design had been ascertained, a USCG design team produced lines for a motor lifeboat based on these. The characteristics of the new lifeboat evolved in July 1960 and a preliminary design was prepared for model tank testing. Self-righting was achieved as a result of the boat's lightweight superstructure, low centre of gravity and hull compartmentation. A 1:12 scale model was constructed from the plans and subjected to resistance and trim tests in the experimental tank of Davidson Laboratory at the Stevens Institute of Technology, Hoboken, New Jersey. This was the first time that a lifeboat design had been model-tested prior to building a prototype. Technology had advanced sufficiently to enable the designers to rely on tests with the model, therby reducing the number of inevitable and costly problems that would appear in a full-scale prototype.

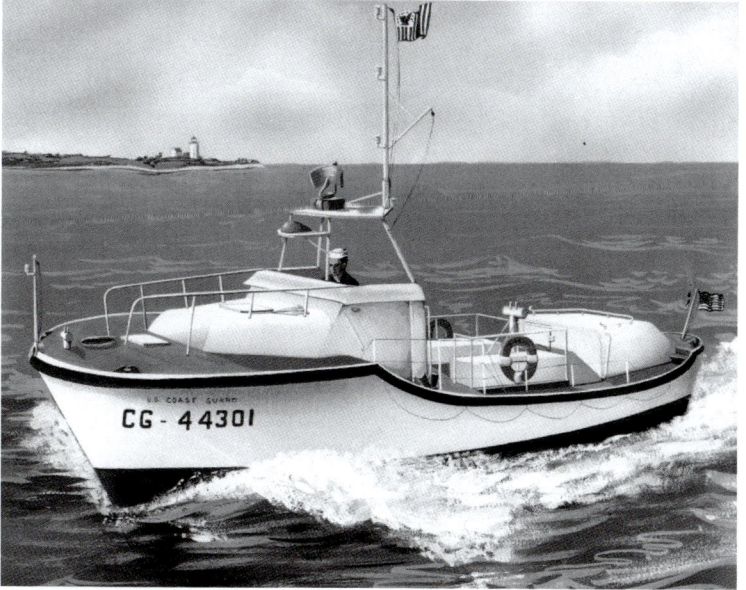

◀ An artist's impression of the USCG 44ft motor lifeboat produced while the design was being finalised. Note the open wheelhouse and minimal electronic aids. The open steering position was probably carried over from the 36-footer but, with its greater speed, the 44-footer needed enhanced crew protection. (USCG photo)

The boat fulfilled its seaworthiness requirements, having the ability to operate in coastal waters under unusually severe weather and sea conditions. It was able to make progress into head seas at speed without damaging to the boat's structure or equipment, and without physically punishing the crew. Not only had it to survive severe sea conditions, but also be able to take the ground, work in heavy surf and tow vessels, while be light enough to achieve a reasonably good speed.

The hull had to combine maximum strength with minimum weight, thus enabling the design to meet the specified criteria. It was constructed from welded Corten steel, a special low carbon formulation possessing high strength and corrosion-resisting properties, which had the benefit of reduced hull maintenance. The bulkheads, hull framing, raised decks and cockpit deck were all constructed of mild steel. To protect the vessel against possible damage should it be grounded, a double bottom was provided in the forward half of the boat, and a strong keel

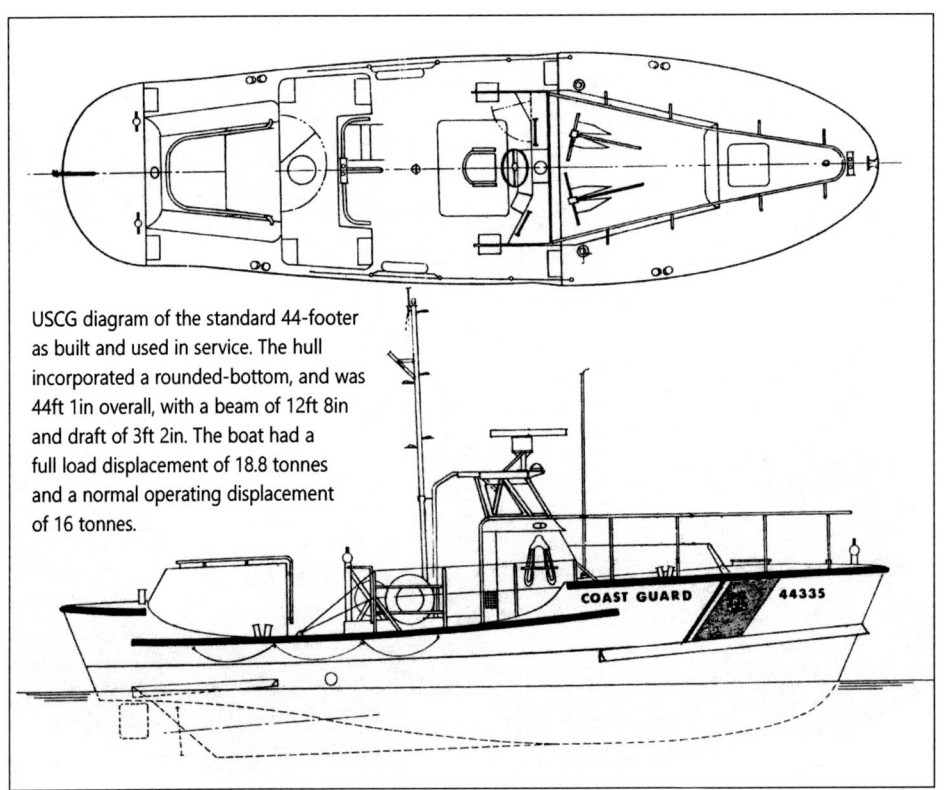

USCG diagram of the standard 44-footer as built and used in service. The hull incorporated a rounded-bottom, and was 44ft 1in overall, with a beam of 12ft 8in and draft of 3ft 2in. The boat had a full load displacement of 18.8 tonnes and a normal operating displacement of 16 tonnes.

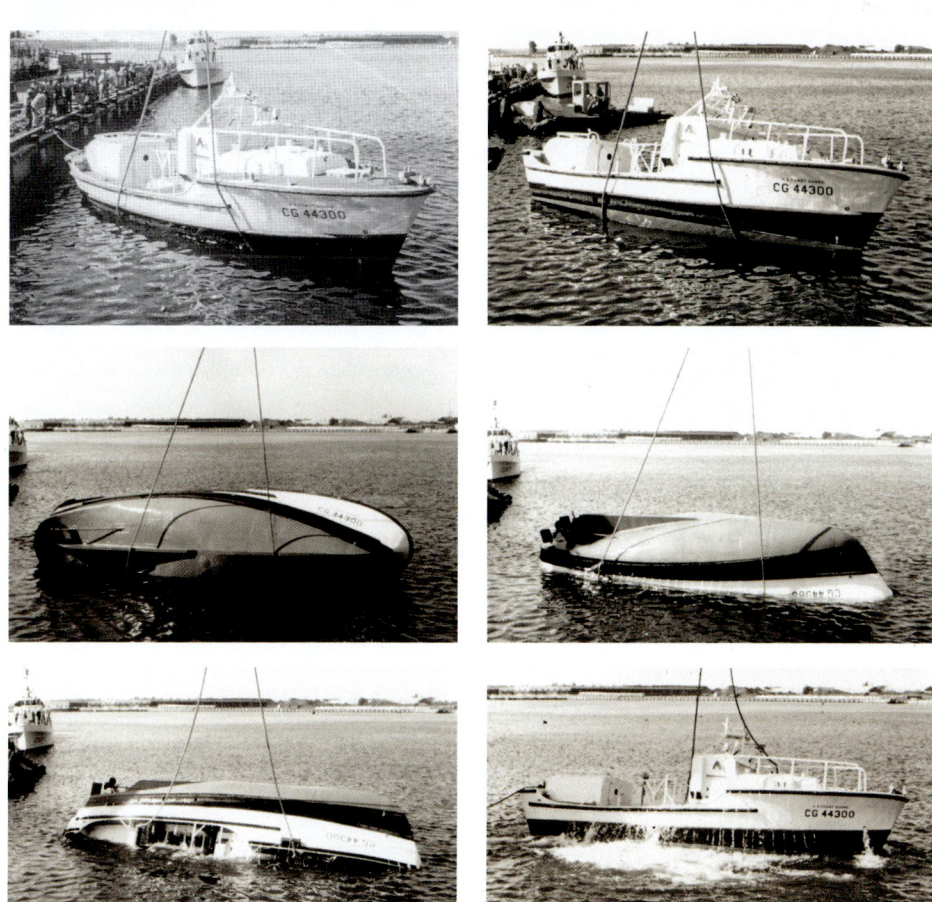

▲ The self-righting characteristics of the 44ft motor lifeboat were tested during capsizing trials. During these trials the boat righted in four to six seconds, depending on whether the fuel tanks were full or not. These photos show the prototype 44-footer CG-44300 being capsized at the USCG yard, Curtis Bay, Baltimore, Maryland on 28 September 1961. (Official USCG photos, courtesy of William Wilkinson)

extended aft. The hull was divided into seven watertight compartments, framed by a combination of transverse and longitudinal bulkheads. The compartments comprised cable locker, forward cabin, crew's cabin, engine room, void space, aft cabin and steering gear compartment.

The open wheelhouse incorporated an adjustable seat for the helm and Morse single lever speed and gearbox controls for operating the main engines. The steering position was also equipped with engine starting controls, an instrument panel, a magnetic compass and remote controls for electronic equipment. Survivor accommodation consisted of seating for ten persons, together with a small galley and toilet. There was stowage space for basic fire-fighting equipment. Towing equipment consisted of a towing bollard four inches in diameter and 100 fathoms (183m) of 28mm diameter nylon rope stowed on a reel with a three-and-a-half-inch circumference.

Power was provided by two 180hp GM 6V-53 diesel engines driving twin three-bladed bronze propellers. The port engine was also used to drive the fire and salvage pump, in addition to the hydraulic system to start the main engines. The starboard engine powered the hydraulic steering pump. After trials of the prototype, stern fins were added just below the water line on either side of the hull to improve the trim of the boat, together with streamlined rudders and power-assisted steering. These modifications greatly enhanced control of the boat and improved its operation when running before a following sea.

The USCG construction programme

Construction of a prototype boat began at the Coast Guard Yard at Baltimore in April 1961 and this was completed in 1962. Designated CG-44300, the new craft was launched in February 1962 and, as the first part of an extended and exhaustive evaluation programme, was subjected to rough water testing on the Atlantic Coast. After initial rough water testing, CG-44300 left the CG Yard on 14 April 1962 and visiting a number of lifeboat stations along the East Coast during a passage from Hatteras Inlet to Maine, before taking up operational duties at Chatham Station, Massachusetts. On 19 October 1962 the boat left Chatham and arrived in Seattle, Washington for evaluation by the 13th Coast Guard District on the north-western coast.

During early November 1962 the boat was tested on the bar at Yaquina

Comparison of characteristics		
	36-footer	**44-footer**
Dimensions	36ft 8in x 10ft 8in	44ft 1in x 12ft 8in
Power	90-100hp (single)	360hp (twin diesels)
Speed	8 knots (approx)	12-15 knots (approx)
Displacement	8.8 long tons	14.2 tons

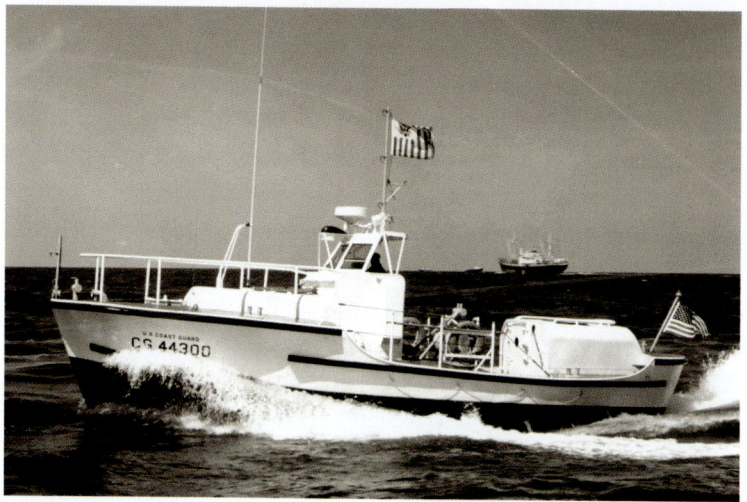

Bay, Oregon, in the heavy breaking surf conditions typical of the Pacific Northwest coast. During the rough-water evaluation, CG-44300 was repeatedly taken into breaking seas on the bar and a nearby reef. With Giles Vanderhoof, a Chief Boatswain's Mate of the USCG, in command, she was brought head-on into the waves. Vanderhoof also turned the stern of the boat to the waves and let the craft be hurled by the heavy breaking seas, which frequently lifted the bow out of the water. Although the impact on its return to the bottom of the intervening trough was considerable, the hull and equipment remained intact.

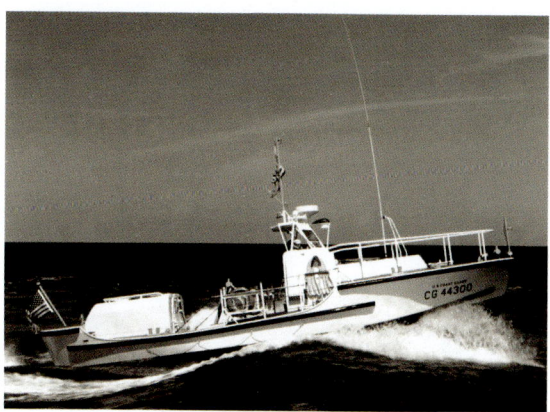

▲ CG-44300 on trials during the early 1960s. The new design gained almost instant approval from the crews who tested her. Power came from twin GM 6V-53 diesels giving a trial speed of 15.3 knots. (Official USCG photos, from the collection of William Wilkinson)

CG-44300 data

Length 44ft 1½in oa, 40ft wl
Beam 12ft 8in oa, 10ft 10in wl
Draft 3ft 2½in
Displacement 15.8 tons
Fuel capacity 333 gallons
Water capacity 16 gallons
Range of stability In excess of 175 degrees
Power Maximum 360hp
Engines Twin GM 6V-53 diesels; twin Cummins V6-200 (production boats)
Trial speed 15.3 knots
Endurance 200 miles at 10 knots, 150 miles at 14 knots

The top of the boat's mast was just over 20ft above the waterline, and the height of the waves was considerably greater than this. Vanderhoof deliberately broached the boat, an almost fatal manoeuvre for small craft, and the breaking seas that engulfed her smashed the windscreen on more than one occasion, but the boat survived. Various items, such as the glass in the windscreen, needed strengthening as a result of the trials, but overall the boat surpassed the expectations of the trials team. Under conditions ranging from large ground swells offshore to short ebb waves, moderate breaking seas and large dangerous seas on bars and reefs, CG-44300 gave excellent performance and survived the trials admirably.

One of the more important design criteria for the 44ft boat was an ability to manoeuvre in the surf, a capability proved during the trials. In taking large breaking seas bow on, the boat had sufficient power which would carry her to the top of the wave to avoid broaching or pitchpoling. Then, just as the bow passed through the top of the break, the power was throttled back and headway lost, so the boat slid down the back of the wave with no pounding experienced. The twin screws, twin rudders and power steering provided an excellent level of manoeuvrability. In the hands of an experienced and skilled Coxswain, the new design could be turned 180 degrees between the crests of two breaking seas,

▼ A 44ft motor lifeboat takes a heavy breaker head-on in conditions typical of the American coasts. (Official USCG photo)

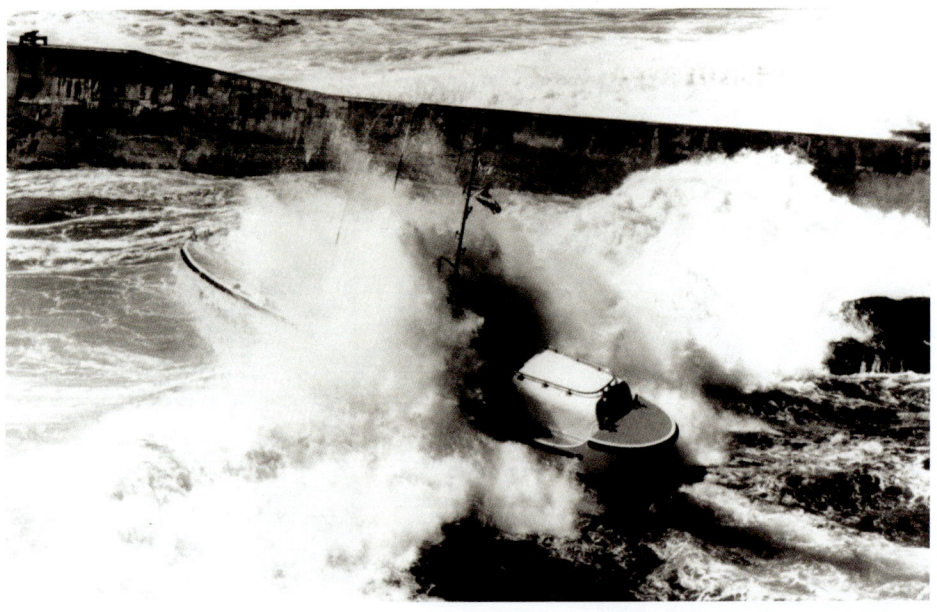

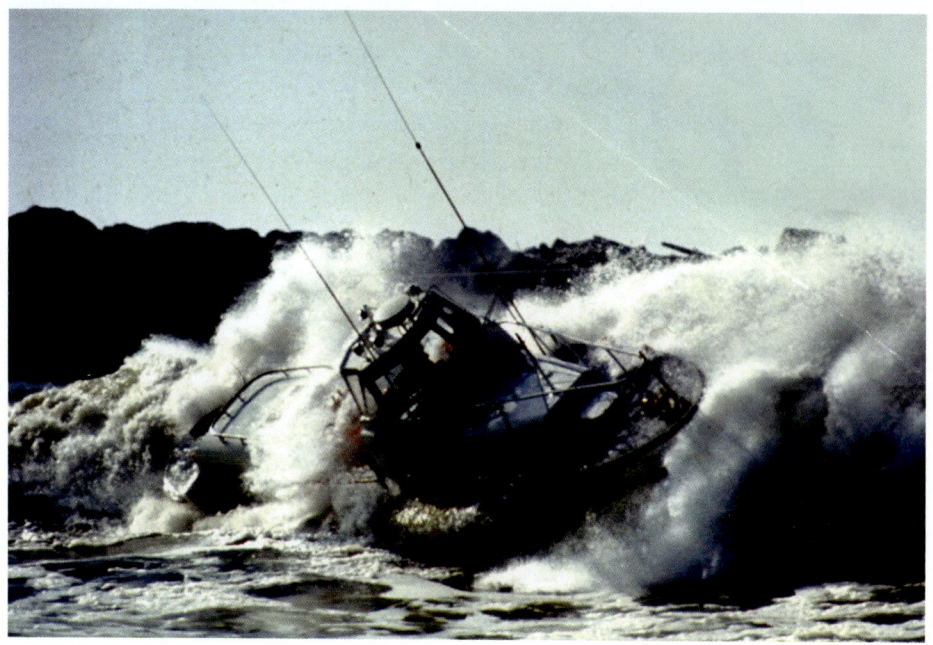

an invaluable capability when taking people from the water in surf conditions. Although various modifications were made as a result of experience gained from the evaluation trials, overall the requirements laid out for the new 44ft design had been fulfilled in the new boat.

During this period CG-44300 cruised approximately 3,000 miles at an average speed of 11.1 knots with a rate of fuel consumption of 20.4 gallons per hour. The boat proved capable of operating up to 50 miles offshore, in surf conditions up to 20 feet, seas up to 30 feet, winds up to fifty knots, and was able to tow vessels up to 125 gross tons. The first serious rescue by CG-44300 took place in December 1962 when, in a south-westerly gale, a 150ft-long barge was towed a distance of eight miles for approximately three hours, in seas up to 15ft in height.

In summary, the outstanding features of the design were identified as follows: strong rudder action and power steering enabling manoeuvres to be quickly executed; exceptional hull design, enabling the boat to negotiate large breaking seas and run into large seas without excessive pounding; crew comfort and safety afforded by good sea-keeping, berthing, padded interiors and adequate compartment heat; a covered steering position giving shelter for the helm; a towing bollard with a

▲ Caught in the surf line, a USCG 44-footer shows the strength and seaworthiness which made her so popular with Coastguardsmen throughout the States. (Official USCG photo)

towing line stowed on an adjacent reel; and hull construction and corrosion protection systems.

Lieutenant Commander Robert Witter, Chief of the USCG Boat Section, stated that 'the all-weather capabilities evidenced throughout this comprehensive development project are considered to rank the USCG 44ft motor lifeboat as one of the finest rescue craft of its type in the world'. The new design was ready to enter service.

In September 1961 Commandant of the Coast Guard, Admiral A.C. Richmond, announced that new 44ft lifeboats would replace 36-footers at the rate of about ten per year. On 9 March 1962 CG Headquarters announced that CG-44300 was to be the prototype for an initial eighteen-boat construction programme, later expanded to twenty-five boats, designated CG-44301 to CG-44324. The long-term intention was to build about 100 44-footers for service at CG rescue stations on the Atlantic Coast from Cape Hatteras north, on the Pacific Coast from San Francisco north, and on the Great Lakes.

Diagrams from the USCG 44ft MLB Type Manual showing some of the equipment used on the 44-footers.

▼ (1) Searchlight; (2) Air horn; (3) Blue light; (4) radar scanner; (5) Mast; (6) VHF radio aerial; (7) VHF automatic radio direction finder aerials (8) AM antenna; (9) 60lb Danforth anchor; (10) 28lb Danforth anchor; (11) bow fairlead; (12) forward mooring bollard; (13) anchor cable hawse pipe. The portable salvage pump (3), towing bollard (1) and tow reel (2) working area, situated aft of the coxswain's position. The midship position of the towing bollard helped to give the 44-footer an excellent towing capability. ▼

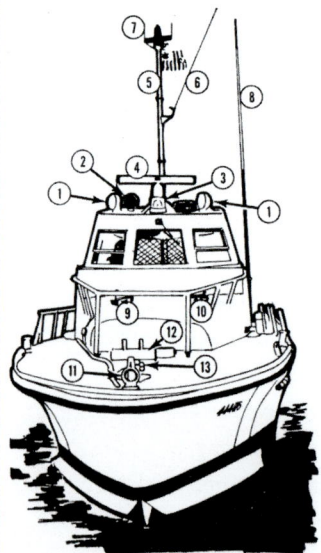

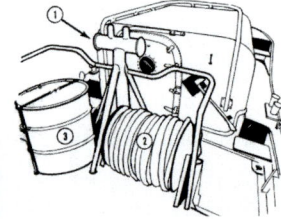

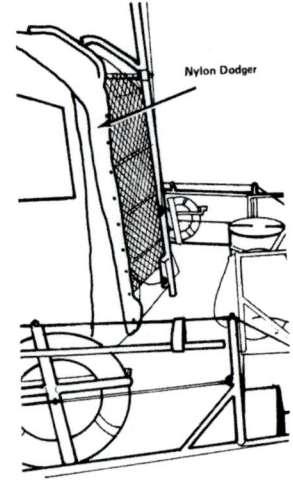
Nylon Dodger

▲ The nylon dodger foul weather curtain attached to the aft portion of the wheelhouse roof helped to protect the coxswain should a wave break over the boat.

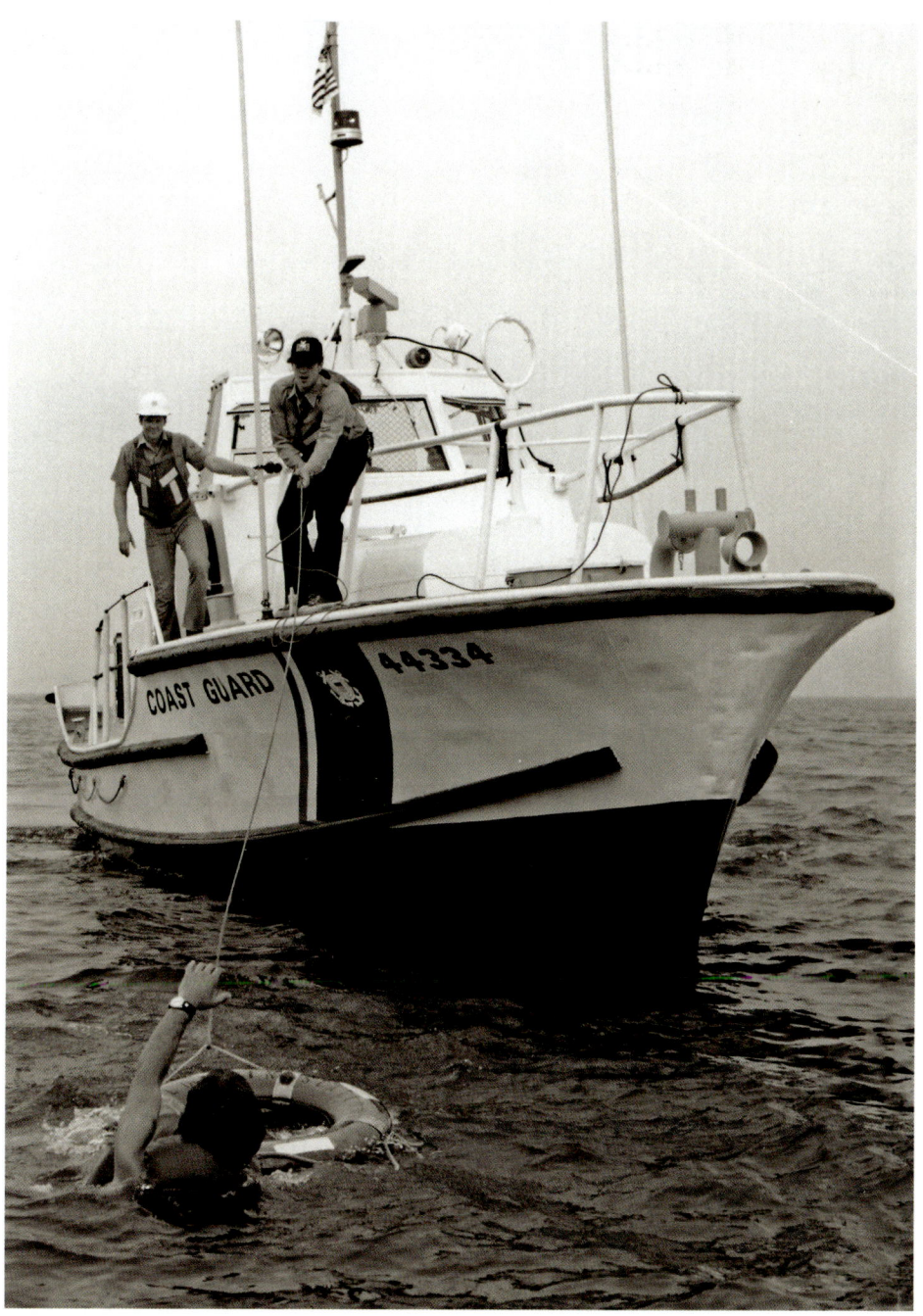

▲ Although primarily used for search and rescue tasks, as illustrated here, 44-footers were also used for law enforcement and other general duties around the coasts of America. (Official USCG photo)

WAVENEY LIFEBOATS

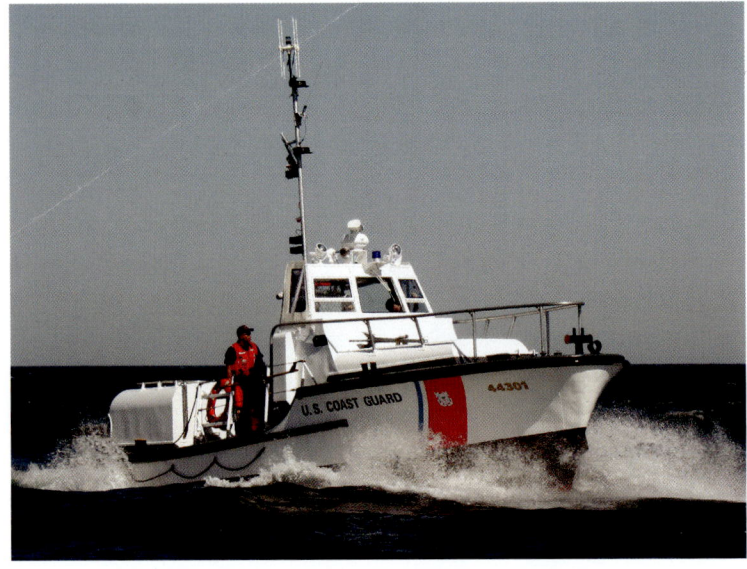

▶ US Coast Guard 44-footer CG-44301 on exercise off Chatham, Massachusetts, September 2006. The boat was taken out of service in 2009 and was placed on static display at Chatham. (Nicholas Leach)

A total of 110 were eventually constructed, of which 106 entered service with the US Coast Guard, while the remaining four were sold for use abroad. All were constructed at the USCG Yard at Curtis Bay, Baltimore, on the Chesapeake River, where one 44-footer could be completed and ready for delivery into service in approximately six months. The boats built in the first construction programme of the 1960s cost $115,000 on average, while the last boat, CG-44409, completed in 1972, cost $225,000. By the 1980s 105 boats were in active service, operating from seventy-seven stations along the Atlantic and Pacific coasts and the Great Lakes.

After the trials had ended, CG-44300 continued in service and between October 1962 and 1981 served at Station Yaquina Bay. In July 1981 she was transferred to the National Motor Lifeboat School at Cape Disappointment, Washington, where she served for a further fifteen years. The boat was often involved in strenuous duties, and was capsized several times during her career. However, she was always up to the task, and won the admiration and affection of her crews, being used to train coxswains and operators from stations throughout the US. The 44-footer became the Coast Guard's standard heavy weather and surf rescue response platform, capable of effecting a rescue at sea under the most difficult circumstances. The outstanding design proved to be almost unsinkable and gained great popularity with Coast Guardsmen.

44ft motor lifeboats for the RNLI

When the RNLI began to show an interest in the USCG 44ft motor lifeboat in 1963, it was the first time the Institution had seriously considered putting a fast lifeboat into service on a nationwide basis. Although a fast lifeboat, 64ft in length and named Sir William Hillary (ON.725), had been built in 1929 for service at Dover, she was essentially a one-off craft and served for only ten years. Designed to attend ditched aircraft in the English Channel, she was powered by twin 375hp engines and could reach speeds of more than seventeen knots. When she was taken over by the Admiralty in October 1940, the RNLI continued to operate a fleet of traditional displacement-hulled double-ended lifeboats until well after World War II.

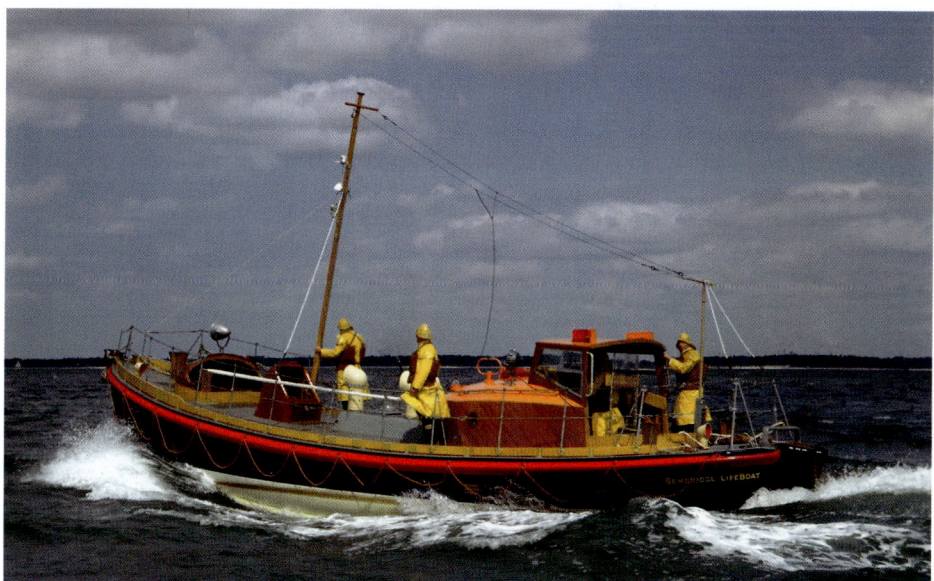

▲ The 46ft Watson Jesse Lumb (ON.822), built in 1939, served at Bembridge for thirty-one years. Not self-righting and with an open aft cockpit, she was typical of the lifeboat designs operated by the RNLI during the first half of the twentieth century, having a wooden hull and a top speed of nine knots. (By courtesy of the RNLI)

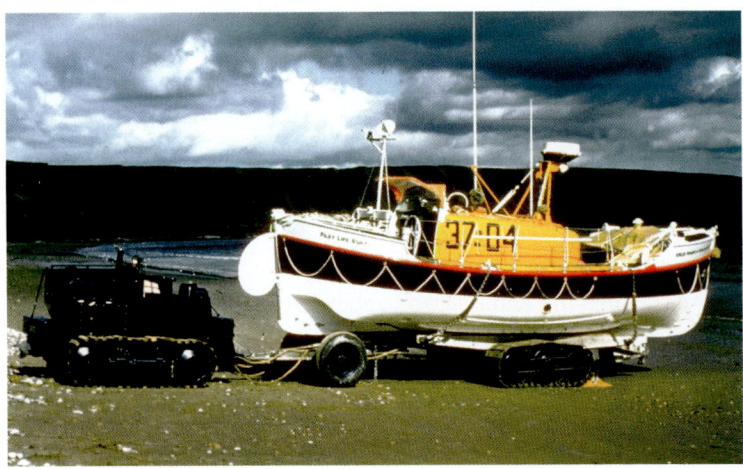

▶ The 37ft Oakley Robert and Dorothy Hardcastle (ON.966) at Filey, on her launching carriage. This Oakley design, when introduced into service in 1958, was seen as a major advance in lifeboat design. It offered both good seakeeping abilities and also a self-righting capability, a combination not achieved before in a British lifeboat design. (By courtesy of the RNLI)

The RNLI's interest in the USCG 44ft lifeboat was therefore a significant development, particularly when seen in the context of post-1945 lifeboat construction in the UK. During World War II the lifeboat service had operated under difficult conditions as lifeboats were forced to work under the guidance of the naval authorities. Moreover, with the country's economy focused on the war effort, fund-raising for charitable causes had been exceptionally difficult. Few new lifeboats had been built and so once peace had been secured the RNLI embarked upon a rapid construction programme. In 1945 the fleet consisted of 151 motor and three pulling lifeboats, so the initial priority was to equip all stations with motor lifeboats, and, between 1945 and 1960, over 100 new motor lifeboats were constructed, an average of eight per annum.

However, these new boats, mostly of the Watson, Barnett and Liverpool types, were based on a nineteenth century hull design, albeit with improved equipment, more powerful engines and twin screws. The broad-beamed non-self-righting designs, which typified British lifeboats up to the 1960s, were first introduced in the 1890s in what was then a radical type of sailing lifeboat. Drawn by George Lennox Watson, the RNLI's Naval Architect, the basic hull shape for non-self-righting lifeboats remained the favoured type around the UK and Ireland until the introduction of the USCG's 44ft design.

Some improvements were implemented in the immediate post-war years, such as the introduction of a midship-steering position in the 46ft 9in Watson class of motor lifeboat, and a policy of fitting all lifeboats with diesel engines was pursued. But the RNLI's position in the 1940s and 1950s was that new and relatively untried ideas and equipment should not be introduced into the lifeboat service. Indeed, in 1947 the RNLI's Chief inspector of Lifeboats, Commander P.E. Vaux, stated that: 'a lifeboat is not the medium to experiment with', and added that every part of a lifeboat should be 'thoroughly tested and proved to the hilt'. Significant technical advances were thus not implemented and the latest technology not employed. Developments and improvements were not groundbreaking.

Although boats based on the displacement hull were fine, seaworthy craft, well suited to rescue work during the first half of the twentieth century, they had two major drawbacks. Firstly, they were not self-righting and, secondly, the hull shape restricted speed to, at best, a little over nine knots irrespective of engine size and power. The first significant advance of the post-war era came during the late 1950s with the introduction of a 37ft lifeboat which overcame the problem of self-righting and was hailed as a major breakthrough. Designed by Richard Oakley, after whom the class was subsequently named, the new design was both inherently stable and also self-righting, a combination that had hitherto eluded lifeboat designers.

Self-righting boats prior to the Oakley type had sacrificed some of their initial stability to achieve self-righting, having a narrow beam, and this meant they were not always popular with volunteer crews.

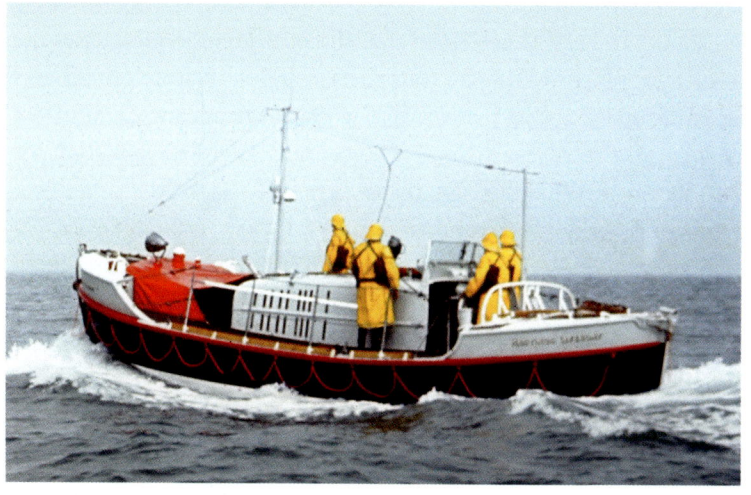

◀ The 37ft Oakley Fairlight (ON.973) on trials off Littlehampton prior to entering service at Hastings. The hull shape was similar to that of the Watsons and Barnetts, and as a result speeds of only about eight knots were possible. (By courtesy of the RNLI)

WAVENEY LIFEBOATS

Oakley's design, however, was self-righting by virtue of a system of water ballast transfer between tanks in the hull, and its hull, which was broad beamed and thus similar to the Watson and Barnett non-self-righting types, provided great stability. However, its displacement hull limited its speed, as this type of hull has to push water out of the way as it moves, creating drag and making it almost impossible to achieve a speed greater than nine knots, and by the 1960s speed had become a factor in life-saving and a faster design was needed.

The International Lifeboat Conference 1963

The breakthrough came after the RNLI hosted the International Lifeboat Conference in Edinburgh between 4 and 6 June 1963. The aim of the International Conferences, held every four years, is to exchange rescue ideas to mutually benefit lifeboat organisations around the world. At Edinburgh, thirty-five papers were read and discussed covering a variety of subjects regarding lifeboats, rescue boat design and life-saving techniques. The RNLI presented papers on first aid in lifeboats, the building of new lifeboat stations at Selsey and Lizard-Cadgwith, and the prototype 48ft 6in Oakley type lifeboat, while delegates from Norway, Sweden, Netherlands and the United States gave papers on newly developed lifeboat designs built in their countries.

The 44ft design intended for general purpose inshore rescue work off the American coasts was described by the USCG delegation, and was of particular interest to several lifeboat institutions, including the RNLI. The USCG explained that the boat was the product of the most comprehensive design, construction and evaluation project ever undertaken for a Coast Guard rescue craft. Lieutenant Commander Witter, of the USCG's Naval Engineering Division, prefaced his description of the design by saying: 'The CG-44300 [the prototype] . . . is considered by this command to be the most remarkable piece of equipment to bolster the operational capabilities of the Coast Guard since the development of the 52-foot MLB'.

With such praise it is hardly surprising that considerable interest was shown by other delegations at the Conference. Although it was not possible to bring one of the new 44-footers to the Conference, a film was shown of the boat in action manoeuvring through the extreme surf

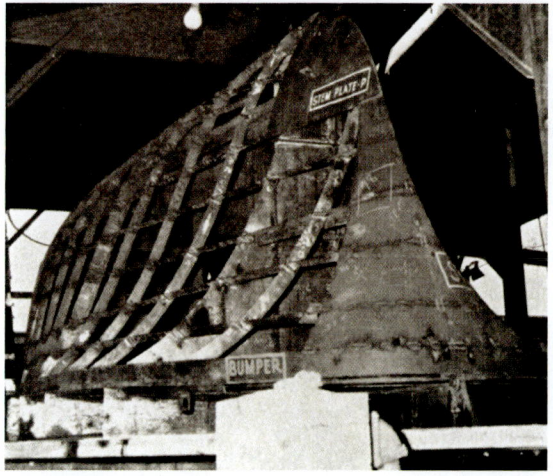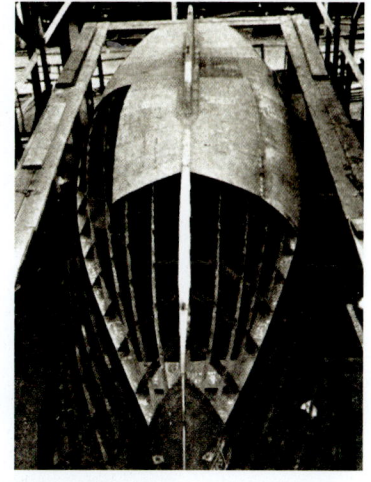

▲ The 44-footer under construction at the US Coast Guard yard at Baltimore, Maryland: the hull was framed by a combination of transverse and longitudinal members, and was divided into seven watertight compartments. A web frame at the mid-section, extending from keel to cockpit deck level, provided protection if the boat grounds.

▼ The 44-footer's steering station was equipped with engine starting and throttle controls, steering wheel, instrument panel, special-damped compass, and remote-operated electronic equipment.

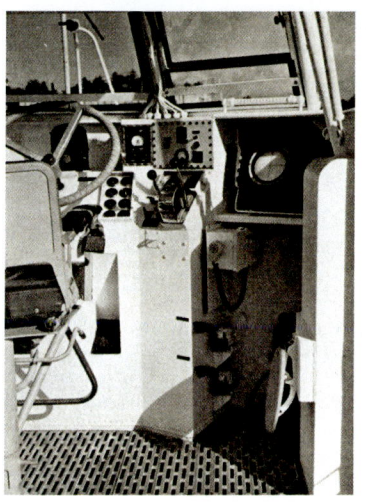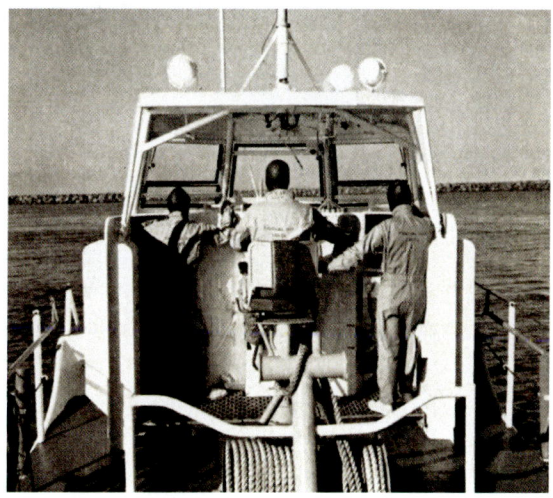

conditions regularly encountered on the Pacific coast. A model was also presented for the delegates to examine. Commander de Booy, Director of the KNZHRM (North and South Netherlands Lifeboat Society), was particularly impressed with what he saw, commenting: 'If you could spare one of these 44ft boats we would like to try her on our coast'.

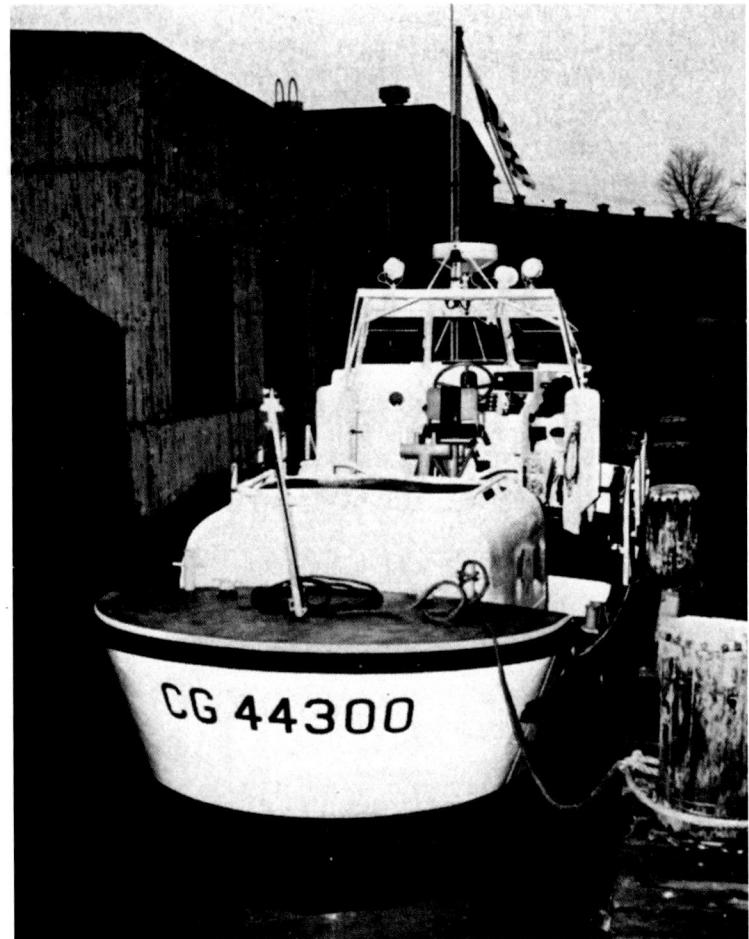

▶ The prototype 44ft motor lifeboat, CG 44300, pictured shortly after her completion in 1962, showing the after deck and stern configuration. This photo accompanied the USCG's paper on the design which was published in the Report on the 1963 International Lifeboat Conference.

CG 44300

The discussion at the Conference covered various areas of the new boat's design and operation. Witter explained that all 44-footers were kept afloat, as the USCG was phasing out launch-ways and boathouses because they were so costly to maintain. He also stated that fitting radar in the steering position was not yet practicable, because the unit must be watertight and such a unit had yet to be found. The question of rudder protection was also raised, but in Witter's view the rudders were well enough protected. He described an incident in which one of the boats was accidentally stranded and driven on to the beach. She was driven off under her own power, and taken back to sea again on the next surf surge, having suffered minimal damage.

The 44ft Waveney enters RNLI service

The RNLI's Conference Delegation in 1963, led by the Right Honourable the Earl Howe, RNVR, then RNLI chairman, was very impressed by the new USCG design and realised that the 44ft motor lifeboat could meet the Institution's initial requirements for a faster rescue boat. After careful consideration by the RNLI's boat and construction committee, the Committee of Management decided that a delegation should be sent to the United States to examine the boat at first hand, and one should be acquired for trials in the UK. Designing a 'fast afloat boat' from scratch was unnecessary when it became apparent to the RNLI that such a craft already existed, and one which had also been tested in extreme conditions on the American coast.

In January 1964 the RNLI delegation, led by Captain the Hon V.M. Wyndham-Quin, visited the United States to inspect USCG craft and in particular the 44ft steel lifeboat. The delegation consisted of

▼ RNLI prototype 44-001, ex-USCG CG-44328, pictured on 13 April 1964 at the US Coast Guard yard, Curtis Bay, shortly after building work had been completed. (Official USCG photo, from the collection of William Wilkinson)

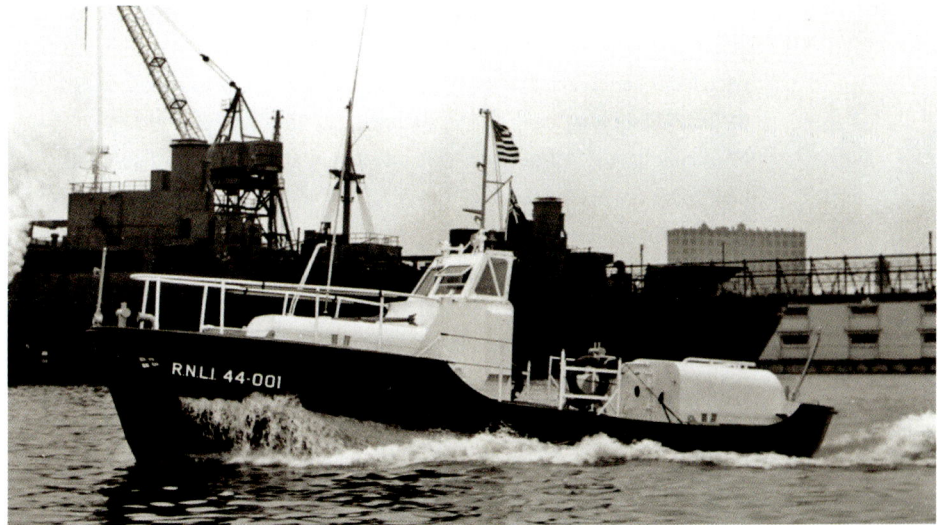

British prototype technical details		
Details of the USCG steel lifeboat compared to the first British-built boat		
	44-001 US prototype supplied to RNLI	44-002 First British-built Waveney
Length	44ft 10½in overall, 40ft waterline	44ft 10½in overall, 40ft waterline
Beam	12ft 8in overall, 10ft 10in waterline	12ft 8in overall, 10ft 10in waterline
Draft	3ft 2½in	3ft 11in
Displacement	15.8 tons	17 tons
Fuel capacity	333 US gallons	350 gallons
Water capacity	16 US gallons	15 gallons
Power (maximum)	400shp (twin Cummins V6 diesels)	430shp (twin Cummins V6 diesels)
Speed (maximum)	15.3 knots (on trials)	14 knots
Endurance	290 miles at 10 knots, 163m at 15 knots	205 miles at 12 knots, 305m at 10 knots
Range of stability	In excess of 175 degrees	180 degrees
Source	The Lifeboat, Vol.38, June 1964, p.67	ILC Report, 1967, Item No.3, p.24

Commander F.R.H. Swann, chairman of the boat and construction committee; Peter Guinness and N. Warrington Smyth, both members of the boat and construction committee; and Lieut-Commander W.L. Gerard Dutton, Chief Inspector of lifeboats, as well as Wyndham-Quin.

After preliminary discussions with USCG officials in Washington, the delegation visited the Coast Guard yard at Curtis Bay, Baltimore, Maryland, and saw a number of the 44ft boats under construction. They also saw other CG craft in action, including an 82ft cutter and amphibious aircraft. An exercise was arranged for the delegation's benefit in which a 44ft motor lifeboat took the 1,300-ton vessel Sassafras in tow. Using a nylon line the lifeboat maintained a speed of nearly six knots, demonstrating that, not only were the 44-footers self-righting and excellent sea boats, but they also had very good towing capabilities.

On returning to London the delegation reported to the Committee of Management, who decided to acquire one of the 44ft vessels for trials. The USCG Commandant agreed to make a fully-equipped boat available for evaluation and service in the United Kingdom, and the 28th boat off the Curtis Bay production line was allocated for RNLI use. After successful sea trials in America with the RNLI's Chief Inspector Lieut-Commander Dutton on board, the boat was accepted by the RNLI and shipped from Baltimore to the United Kingdom by sea as deck cargo.

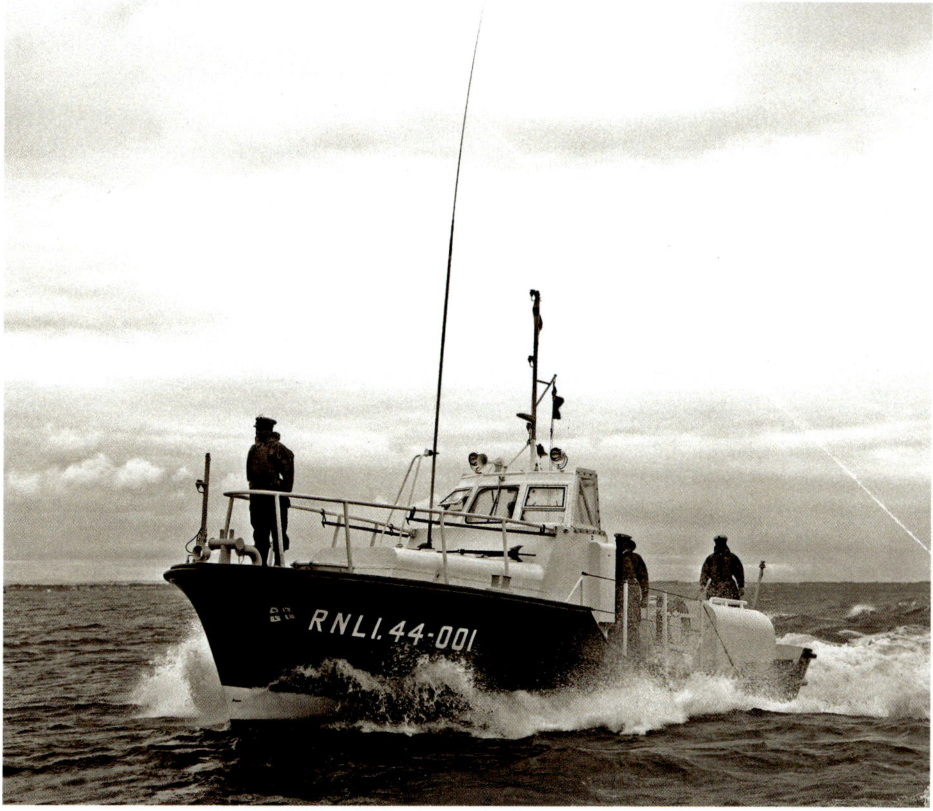

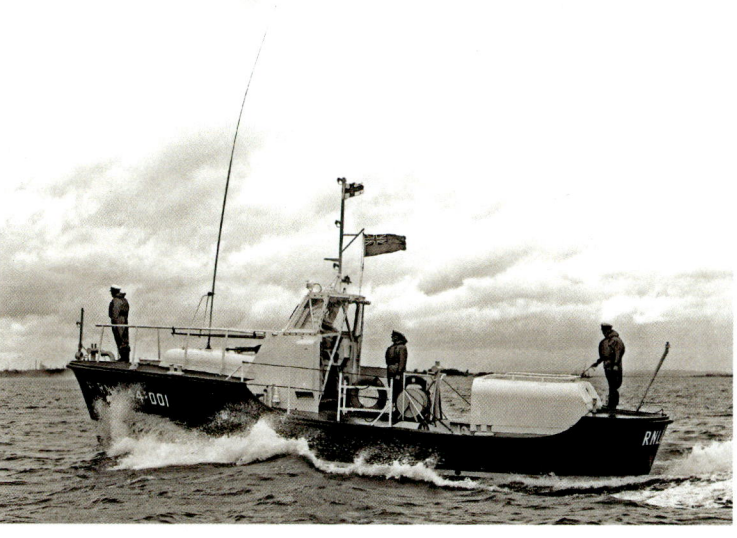

▲ The RNLI's prototype 44ft motor lifeboat was designated 44-001, having been built by the USCG in Curtis Bay, Maryland. She is pictured off Cowes on 15 September 1964 during her initial trials. (Beken, by courtesy of the RNLI)

The boat arrived in London in May 1964 and became the prototype vessel, numbered 44-001 by the RNLI. She then commenced extensive trials around the coasts of Great Britain and Ireland. In December 1964 trials were carried out off the Dutch coast in association with the Royal South Holland Lifeboat Society (KZHMRS), which had also expressed interest in the boat at the 1963 Conference. 44-001 was then subjected to further trials at lifeboat stations and used to train crews to handle the then unique boat. The last stages of the trials were carried out off the coasts of Scotland and north-east England, after which 44-001 was taken south. The initial evaluation period lasted until September 1965, during which time 44-001 covered nearly 5,000 miles.

Construction of the 44-footers in Britain

At the time of the trials of the USCG design, no RNLI lifeboat was capable of a speed greater than nine knots. The speed of the new 44ft lifeboat was achieved by the semi-planing hull design, unlike traditional British lifeboat designs which were based around a displacement double-ended hull form. Semi-planing hulls lift out of the water when a certain speed is reached, reducing the drag of the hull, and thus enabling a greater speed to be achieved. The 44-footer's hull shape was therefore a radical departure from previous British lifeboat designs.

Being so different from any serving RNLI lifeboat type, 44-001 was initially something of a curiosity to lifeboat crews when they saw her

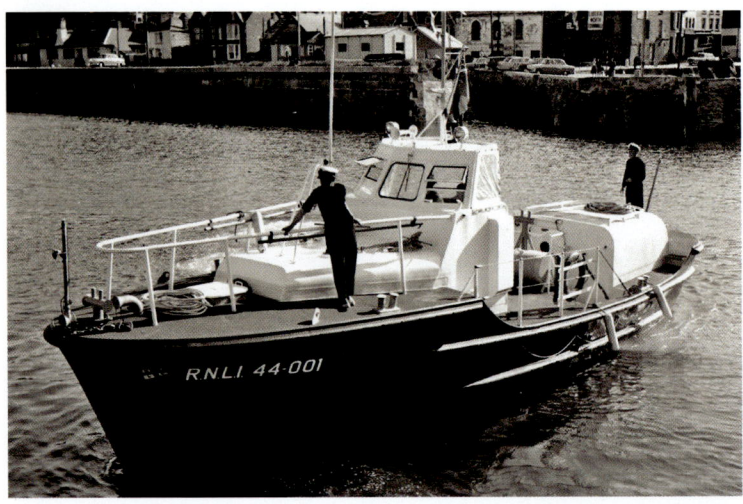

▶ 44-001 at Padstow in 1964 during her evaluation trials around the United Kingdom and Ireland. (By courtesy of the RNLI)

ALTERATIONS AND ADDITIONS BY THE RNLI

1 Aluminium alloy main deck, in place of steel.

2 After cabin increased in height by 2in and coachroof forward of steering shelter increased in volume to improve SR ability.

3 Increased weather protection for helmsman by fitting permanent sides and windows to the wheelhouse, in place of portable screens.

4 Bolted A brackets in place of welded P brackets.

5 Hydraulic pump for windlass fitted in place of hand anchor recovery.

6 Two 65lb anchors fitted, in place of one 60lb and one 30lb.

7 Pushpit rails fitted to raised deck aft.

8 Mathway mechanical steering gear fitted, in place of hydraulic gear.

9 Foam-filled double-bottom fitted in engine room. Foam also filled forepeak, port and starboard at after end of cabin and in centre section of the void space below the well deck for buoyancy in case of hull damage.

10 Reserve fuel tank fitted between frame 4 and 5.

11 Engine room ventilators draw air from inside the steering position, to prevent spray from entering the engine room.

12 Wave subduing oil system fitted.

13 Battery boxes recessed into tank top in crew's cabin.

14 Windscreen washing system fitted.

15 Port and starboard navigation lights fitted in screens on wheelhouse top.

16 Natural ventilation system fitted to after cabin with RNLI design inlet and outlet valves.

17 Toilet compartment removed, and this space fitted out as radio operator's area.

18 RNLI duplex scuppers fitted in both wells in addition to the ball valves.

19 Ford Mermaid engines of 250bhp (various engines were used at different times; see p.4).

20 Auxiliary diesel generator fitted for battery charging.

21 Two fire hydrants and one fire and two bilge pumps driven by main engines, in place of one hydrant and one pump with one engine room bilge eductor.

22 Fixed bilge suctions fitted in engine room.

23 Water injected stern exhausts, in place of transverse exhausts.

24 Electrical distribution by double pole circuit breakers.

25 Engine room fire extinguishing system operated from the wheelhouse.

26 D/F and Decca Navigator installed.

27 Intercom system with master unit in wheelhouse serving after cabin, crew's cabin, forward cabin and fore deck.

28 Depth recorder fitted in crew's cabin in addition to indicator in wheelhouse.

29 Transmission and reception of M/F radio from wheelhouse in addition to radio operator's position.

30 Single whip aerial on the forward casing replaced by two whip aerials on wheelhouse.

at first hand during the trials. However, the trials were deemed very successful, as the boat proved capable of operating in all conditions that were encountered around the British Isles, as a result of which the RNLI decided to build six boats to the design. From the documents put at the RNLI's disposal by the USCG, specifications and comprehensive drawings were prepared. Where possible British materials were specified by the RNLI, as were British components and equipment, with the exception of the main engines and a small number of minor items, so that construction in Britain could be readily undertaken.

The RNLI made a number of changes to the original US design. These included fitting an additional fuel tank, constructing a double bottom beneath the machinery compartment, and extending the wheelhouse to improve crew protection. Raised forward and aft cabin tops improved the self-righting ability, and an additional power take-off on the starboard engine powered a hydraulic pump unit to operate the windlass.

The hull was constructed from Corten corrosion-resistant steel because it was decided at the outset that the vessel should be kept as near as possible to the original USCG design. However, the main deck plating and wheelhouse were constructed of aluminium alloy, rather than steel as was the case with the USCG's boats. These modifications were not carried out retrospectively on 44-001, which therefore remained different from the British-built boats.

In the summer of 1965 tenders were invited for building six boats to the new design. The contract for the work was awarded to the Lowestoft firm of Brooke Marine Ltd, which began construction towards the end

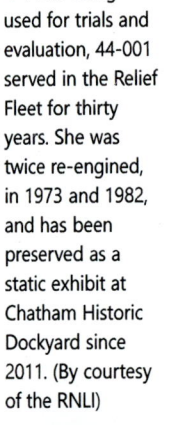

▼ After being used for trials and evaluation, 44-001 served in the Relief Fleet for thirty years. She was twice re-engined, in 1973 and 1982, and has been preserved as a static exhibit at Chatham Historic Dockyard since 2011. (By courtesy of the RNLI)

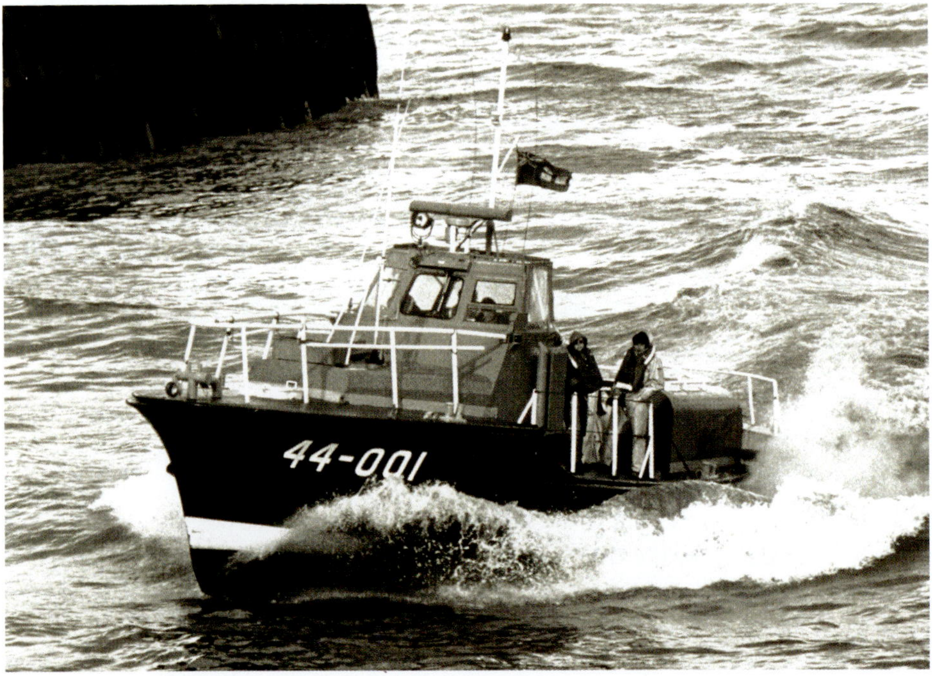

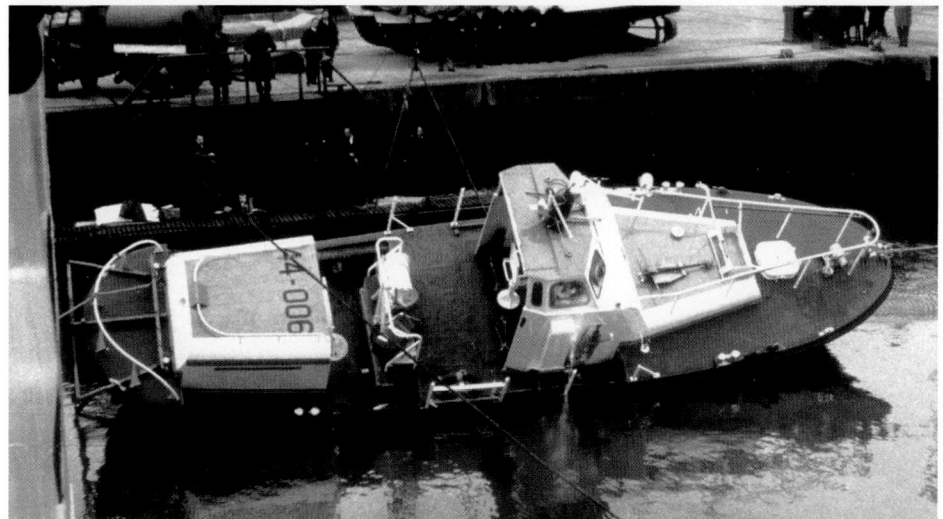

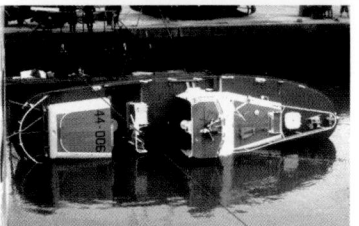
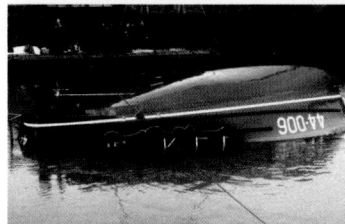

Self-righting trials of 44-006 at Lowestoft in 1968, with the boat being hauled over, then righting herself. (By courtesy of the RNLI)

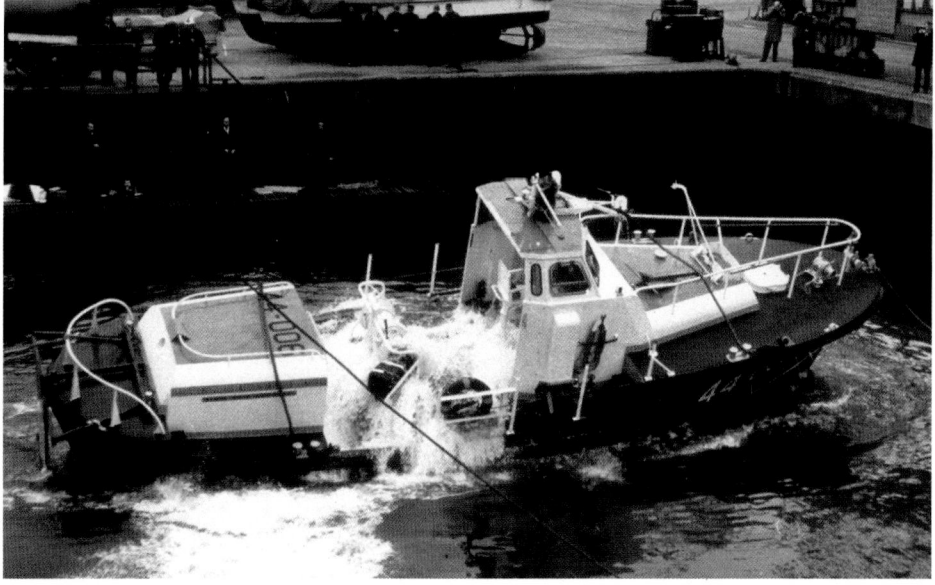

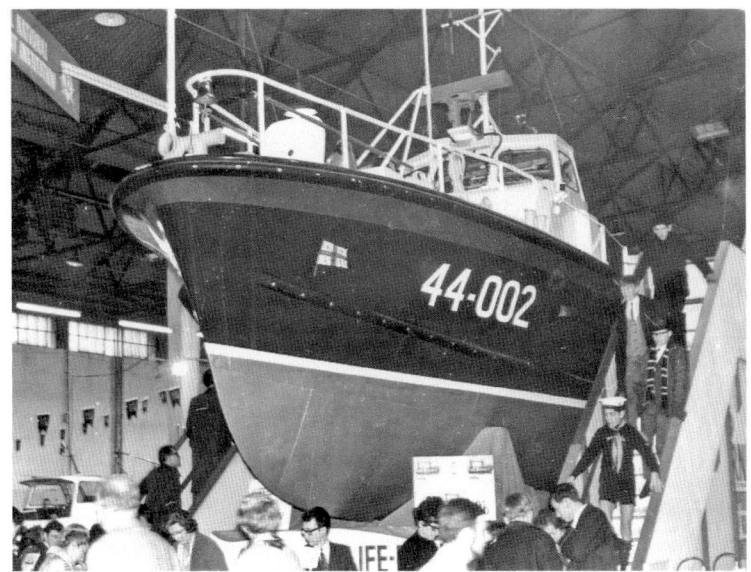

of 1965. The first boat was completed thirty-six weeks after the RNLI had placed the order, and the total cost of the new boats was approximately £158,700. As the boatyard which built these first six boats was situated on the river Waveney, the type was given the class name Waveney in 1972, when the RNLI started its policy of naming lifeboat classes after rivers; Arun, Thames, Rother, Clyde, Brede and Tyne have followed.

The first seven Waveneys (including 44-001) were built with Cummins main engines, model V6N215M, giving a speed of thirteen knots. The first six British-built boats were fitted with a reverse and 3:1 reduction gearbox, type 76/100, made by the Parsons Engineering Co Ltd, of Southampton. The next eight boats (44-008 to 44-015) were built with General Motors diesels, and the remainder had either Ford Mermaid or Caterpillar diesels. The earlier boats were subsequently re-engined with Caterpillar diesels. 44-001 steamed in excess of 5,000 hours on her original Cummins type V200 engines. During 1974 she was re-engined with Ford Mermaid 595 turbo-plus units developing 250bhp each, which gave her a speed of sixteen knots, before subsequently being fitted with Caterpillar engines.

A variety of electronic equipment, different from that in the US boats, was installed and upgraded over time as improved models became available. Initially, the electronic equipment comprised a Kelvin Hughes Type 17 radar, with a watertight display unit in the wheelhouse; Redifon

The third RNLI 44ft Waveney Faithful Forester (44-004) on station at Dover during the early years of her career. (Grahame Farr, by courtesy of the RNLI)

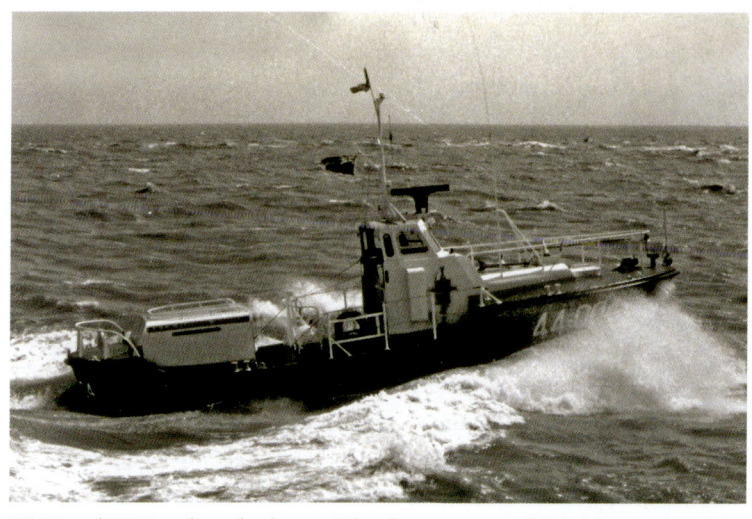

UHF and VHF radio telephone; Woodsons type 90 MF radio equipment; and a Ferrograph combined echo sounder unit. The deckheads and sides of the boat throughout the accommodation were lined with plastic heat and sound insulation foam. All exterior and some interior steelwork was shot blasted prior to painting.

The designated number of crew on the Waveney was five, but often six or seven would be taken on service. Crew comfort was minimal. The

The sixth RNLI Waveney, Connel Elizabeth Cargill (44-007), on trials off Lowestoft shortly after being built. She served at Troon for seventeen years, before stints at Arklow and Portree.

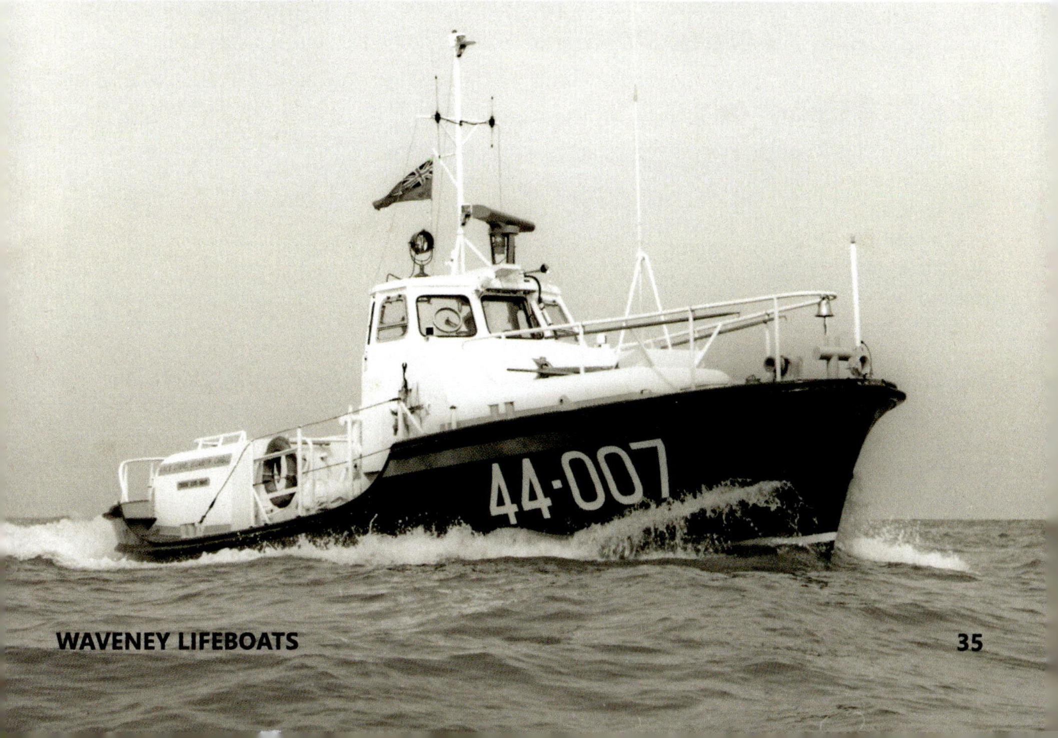

Coxswain was seated in an open wheelhouse that offered only limited shelter, while those standing near the door to the aft cabin could get wet in anything other than benign conditions. Seats were provided for the crew in the cabin, but it was common for them to remain on deck, usually standing behind the wheelhouse. During the boats' careers canvas screens were fitted across the rear of the wheelhouse to offer some shelter, but the wheelhouses were never fully enclosed. The forward cabin was fitted with a bench seat in the crew compartment and limited galley facilities, forward of which was a passenger compartment. The aft cabin had seating for survivors and space for a stretcher.

Some RNLI crews were initially disconcerted by the design's apparently low stability, caused by the hull shape. However, the boats' general behaviour, seaworthiness and high power, which enabled them to pull clear of dangerous situations, soon endeared them to crews around the coasts. The Waveney was so different from the RNLI lifeboats then in service that it was natural for crews to treat it with an initial degree of suspicion. However, as Troon Coxswain Ian Johnson found, the boats were 'highly manoeuvrable, great for towing, and although they were a bit lively at sea, they proved their worth many times over in difficult situations'.

The first six RNLI 44ft Waveneys, which were built by Brooke Marine, were allocated to Dun Laoghaire, Great Yarmouth & Gorleston, Dover, Harwich, Barry Dock and Troon. The first to enter service was John F. Kennedy (44-002), which was placed on station at Dun Laoghaire in May 1967, covering the waters of Dublin Bay and the Irish Sea. The

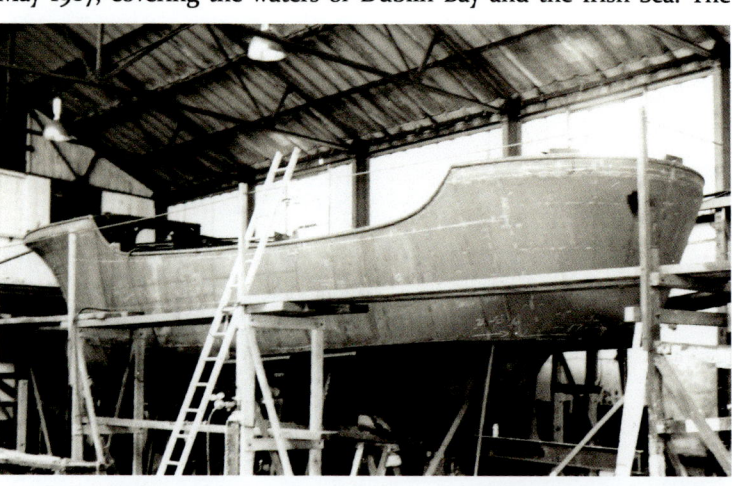

▶ The seventh Waveney to be built by the RNLI, ON.1026 (44-008), allocated to Eyemouth, under construction at Groves & Guttridge boatyard at Cowes, IOW, July 1972. She was the first of the second batch of Waveneys to be built. (Jeff Morris)

WAVENEY LIFEBOATS

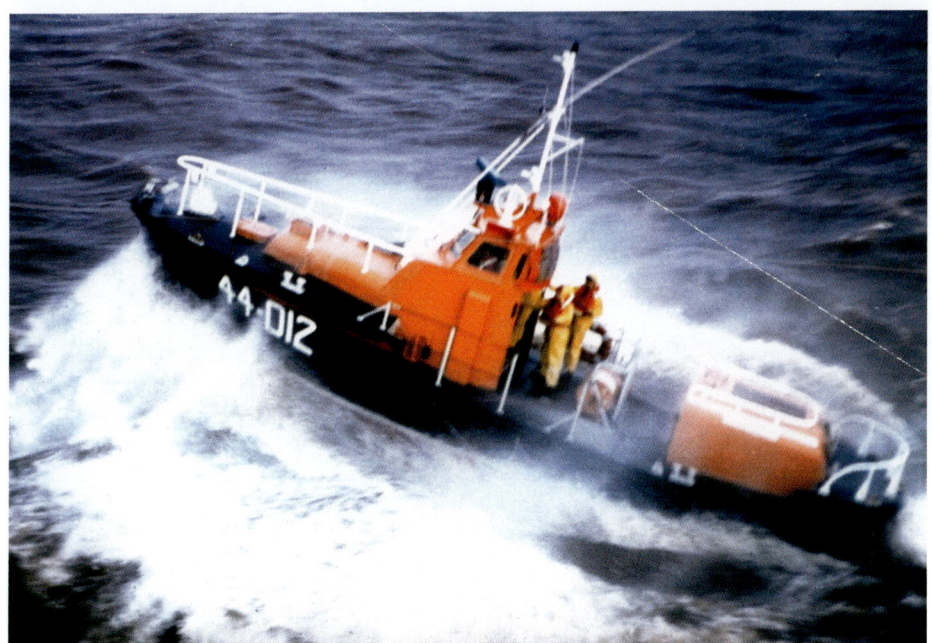

next four boats all entered service in 1967, with the sixth going to Barry Dock in March 1968, and the last, 44-007 for Troon, taking up duties in August 1968. The prototype, 44-001, acted as a relief lifeboat for those on station. These first six boats were sent to different parts of the country to assess the suitability of the design in differing sea conditions, and to stations where a fast lifeboat was deemed particularly beneficial. For example, Barry Dock covered the Bristol Channel following the withdrawal of the 37ft Oakley at neighbouring Weston, while Troon needed a fast lifeboat because of concerns over possible ditched aircraft from the nearby Prestwick airport.

The next batch of Waveneys was not ordered until the early 1970s, with construction of four more boats at the Cowes boatyard of Groves & Guttridge. These four, all of which entered service in 1974, were fitted with more powerful General Motors diesels, each of 260hp as opposed to the 215hp of the Cummins engines in the original six boats. The Cummins engines had proved problematic in service conditions, with the hydraulic starter not proving ideal. Indeed, the Americans changed their hydraulic starters for electric in 1968. The GM engines had an electric starter, which was more reliable, and the engines offered

▲ White Rose of Yorkshire (44-012) in heavy seas off Whitby. She was one of the eight Waveneys built at Cowes by Groves & Guttridge. (By courtesy of the RNLI)

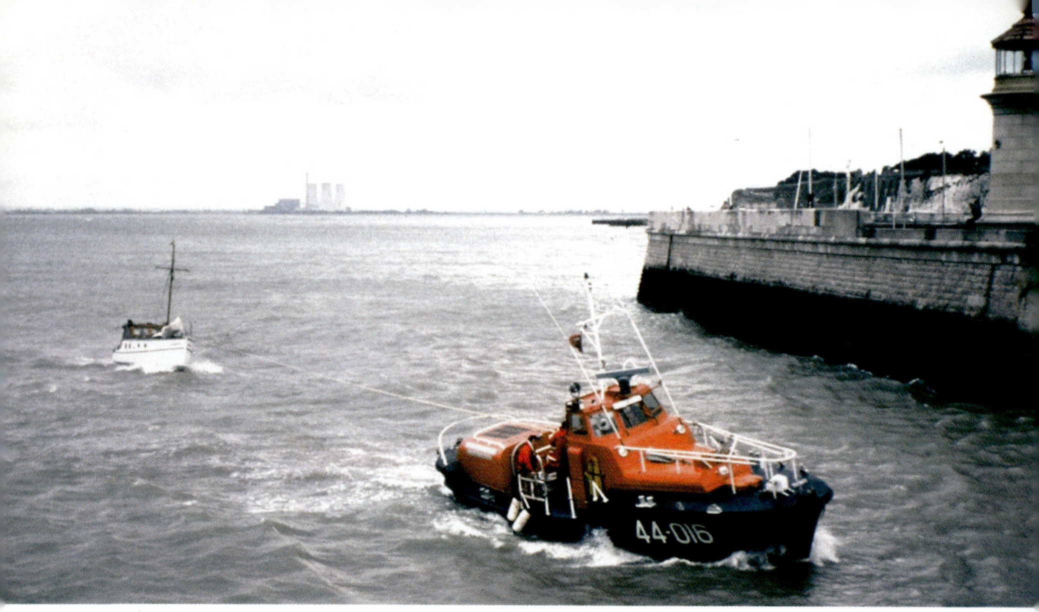

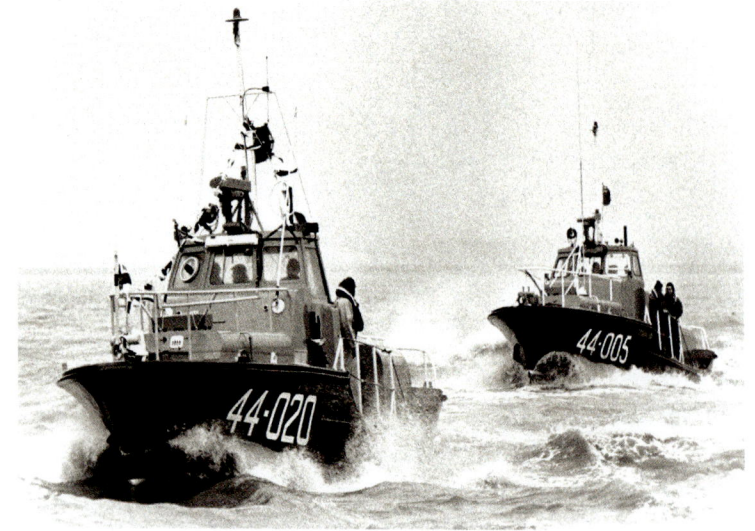

Swann (44-016)
towing a broken
down motor boat
into Ramsgate
Harbour. She was
one of the four
Waveneys built in
North Devon by
Bideford Shipyard.
(By courtesy of
the RNLI)

better performance, so the boats fitted with these were slightly faster. The first of this second batch, 44-008, arrived at Eyemouth in the Scottish Borders in February 1974 and the last, 44-011, reached Poole in November that year.

A second batch of four GM-powered boats was ordered from Groves & Guttridge before the Cowes yard had finished its original four and these next four boats all entered service in 1975. The first, 44-012, went to Whitby, and the last, 44-015 to Fleetwood. With the RNLI now intent

▶ John Fison
(44-020) leads
Margaret Graham
(44-005) into
Harwich in March
1980 to take over
station duties. John
Fison was one
of the last three
Waveneys to be
built, all of which
were completed
by Fairey Allday
Marine at Cowes.

WAVENEY LIFEBOATS

Sectional drawing of 44ft Waveney

Key to the numbers in the drawing as follows: (1) Fairlead, (92) Bollard, (3) Emergency Tiller Cap, (4) Steering Gear, (5) Locker Seat, (6) Stern Floodlight, (7) Grab Rail, (8) Stokes Stretcher, (9) Main Engines, (10) 5-gallon Foam Cans, (11) Quick Acting Watertight Doors, (12) Exhaust Outlet, (13) Engine Exhaust Silencer, (14) Towing Bollard, (15) Breeches Buoy, (16) Steering Transmission, (17) Console, (18) Compass, (19) radar Display Unit, (20) Helmsman's Seat, (21) Engine Room Ventilation Trunking, (22) Ship's Bell, (23) Stern Light, (24) Searchlight, (25) Towing Light, (26) UHF Dipole Aerial, (27) Masthead Light, (28) Radar Scanner, (29) Straight Line Windscreen Wiper, (30) 60lb Danforth Anchor, (31) Chemical Toilet, (32) Radio Telephones, (33) Lifting Eyeplate, (34) Whip Aerial, (35) Boat Hook, (36) Watertight Hatch, (37) Echo Sounder, (38) Hydraulic Windlass, (39) Stemhead Fairlead and Jackstaff Socket, (40) Anchor Light.

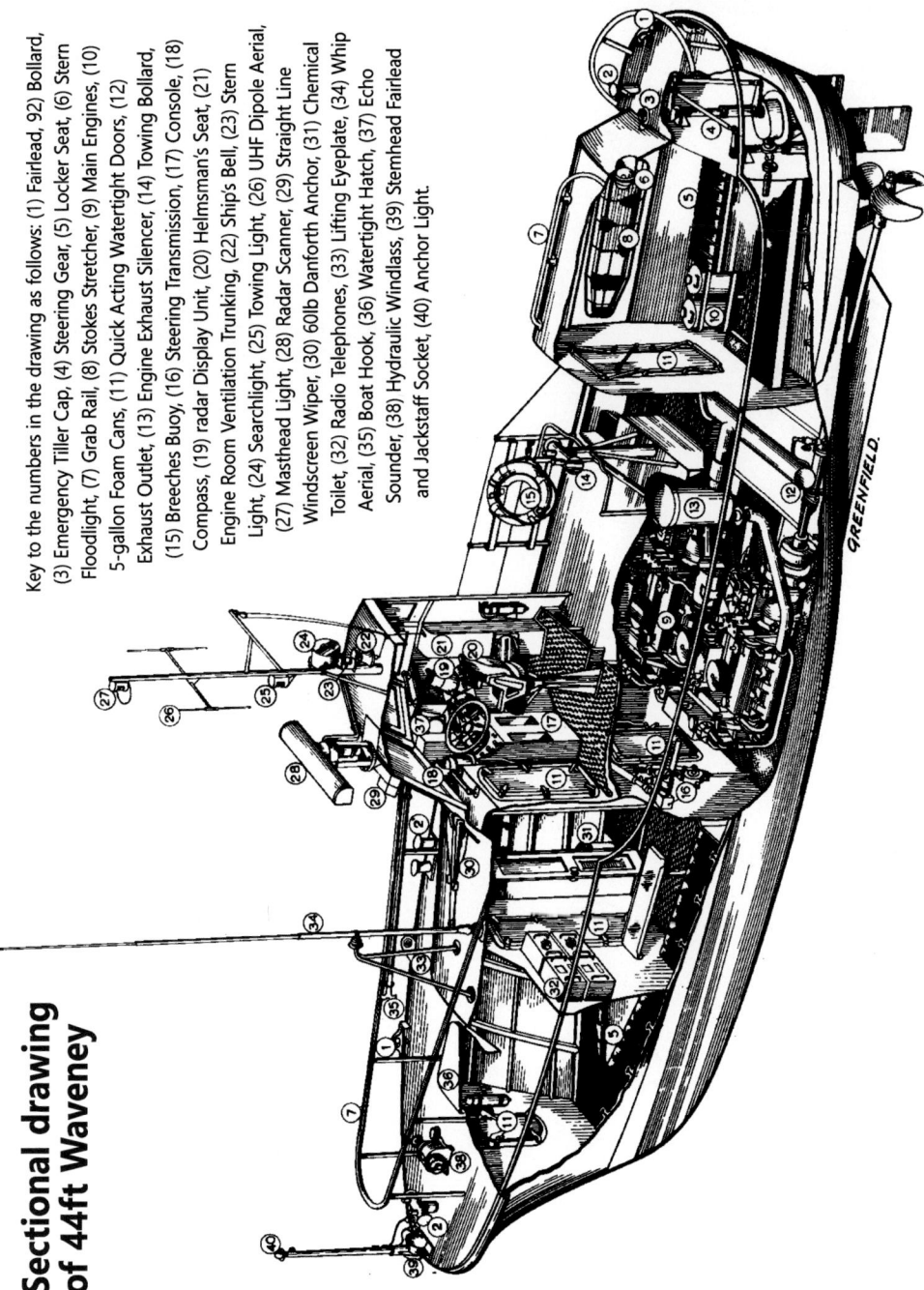

GREENFIELD.

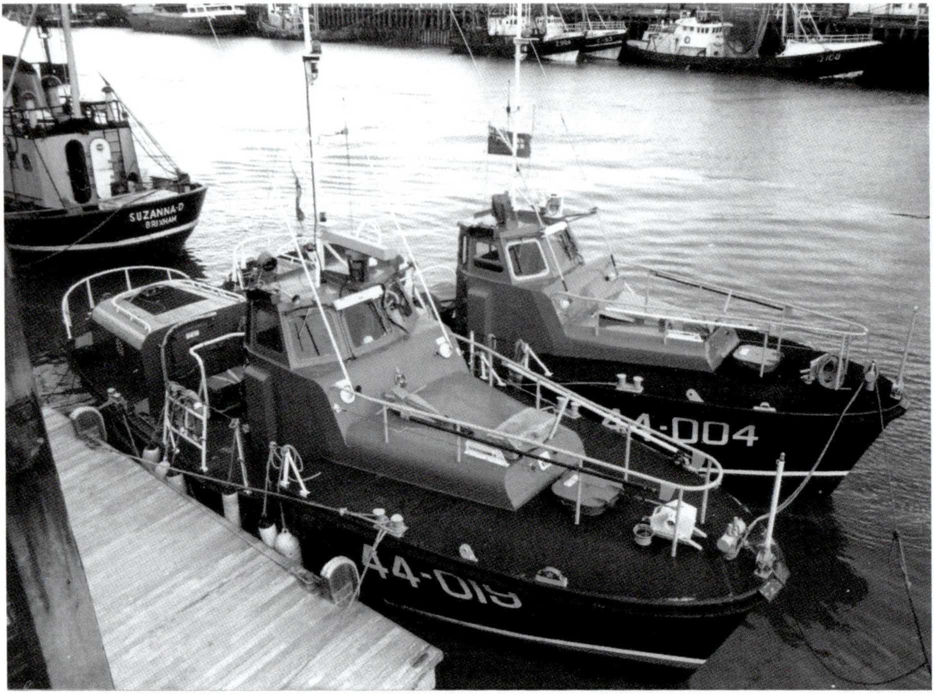

WAVENEY LIFEBOATS

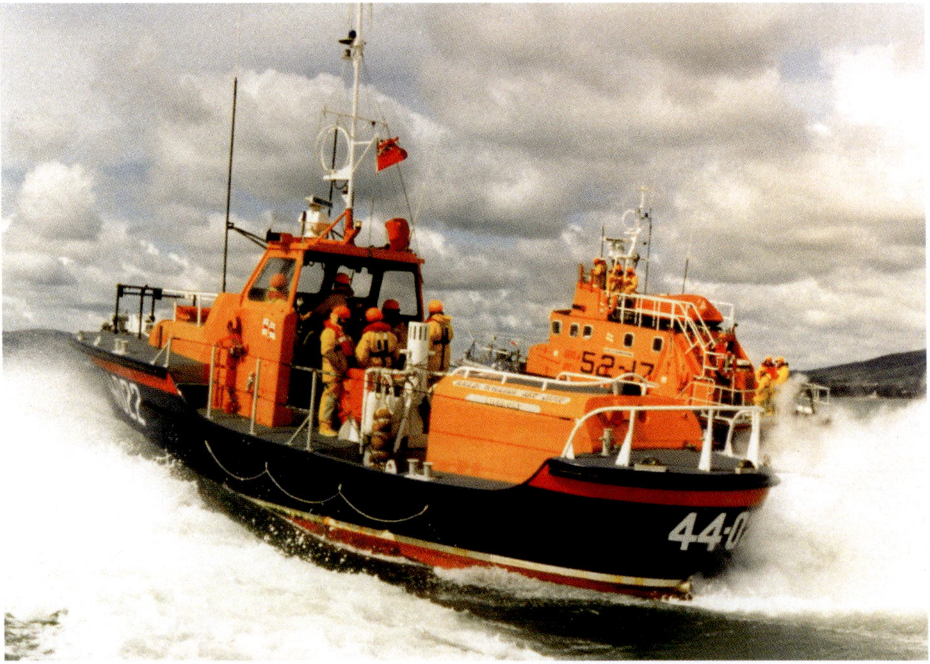

on building a fleet of fast self-righting lifeboats, the Waveneys were an integral part of this plan. A further four Waveneys, 44-016 to 44-019, were ordered from the Bideford Shipyard in North Devon, and entered service in 1976-77. They were powered by Ford Mermaid diesels, but these were found to be unreliable and within less than five years of these four boats entering service each had been re-engined with Caterpillar D3208T diesels. The last three Waveneys were built by Fairey Allday Marine at Cowes: two were completed in 1980, and the last in 1982.

Worldwide service

The success with which the 44ft design had been adapted for use in Britain demonstrated to other sea rescue organisations the possibilities it offered. Well suited to a wide variety of sea conditions, the 44ft design has been used extensively throughout the world. Interest came from the USCG's neighbours in Canada, and in 1966 the Canadian Government bought one for use by the recently formed Canadian Coast Guard (CCG). On 14 September 1966 a USCG-built 44-footer was loaded on board the ice-breaking ship Edward Cornwallis and taken to Canada. This first CCG 44-footer went into service at Clark's Harbour, Nova Scotia in 1966, with Canadian-built versions following, serving on the country's east and west coasts. They were given a red hull, but the livery of the superstructure altered between white and SAR yellow. All the Canadian 44-footers had enclosed wheelhouses, which some crew found to be rather claustrophobic. However, as in Britain and the United States, the boats served with distinction, with the last being replaced in 2004 when the CCGC Souris departed its Prince Edward Island base.

In Europe, Norway, Portugal and Italy have all used the 44ft design. In 1968 two 44ft boats entered service with the Norwegian Sea Rescue Society, designated R/S 73 and R/S 74 and named Ole O. Hoshovde and Arne Fahlstrøm respectively. They operated in Norway until the mid-1970s having had the wheelhouse enclosed to enable the crews to operate them in the extreme cold experienced in Norwegian waters.

The 44ft design was also used by the Italian Coast Guard, which purchased two boats from the USCG, one of which served until April 2000 and has been on display in front of the headquarters of the Ravenna Captaincy in Porto Corsini. Two 44-footers were also used by

◀◀ Two Waveneys at Newhaven: station boat Louis Marchesi of Round Table (44-019), nearest camera, and relief lifeboat Faithful Forester (44-004) alongside. 44-019 was the last of the four Waveneys built by Bideford Shipyard in North Devon. After her time at Newhaven, she served at Alderney for almost eight years and then Exmouth for two years. (By courtesy of Roger Cohen)

◀◀ The last Waveney in service in Ireland, The William and Jane, at Larne in 1988, just prior to being replaced by the 52ft Arun Hyman Winstone (ON.1067). (By courtesy of the RNLI)

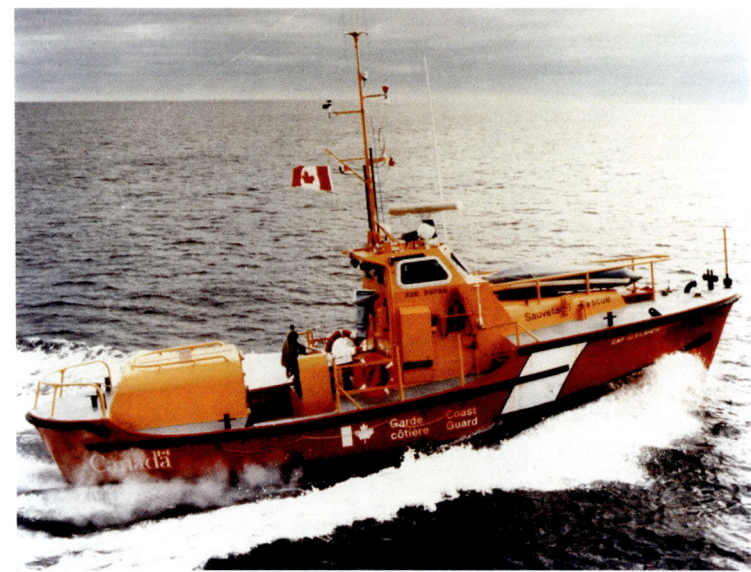

◢ Canadian Coast Guard 44ft Type 300 lifeboat CCGC Cap Goélands was built in 1985 at Hike Metal Products Ltd, Wheatley, Ontario, based on the USCG design.

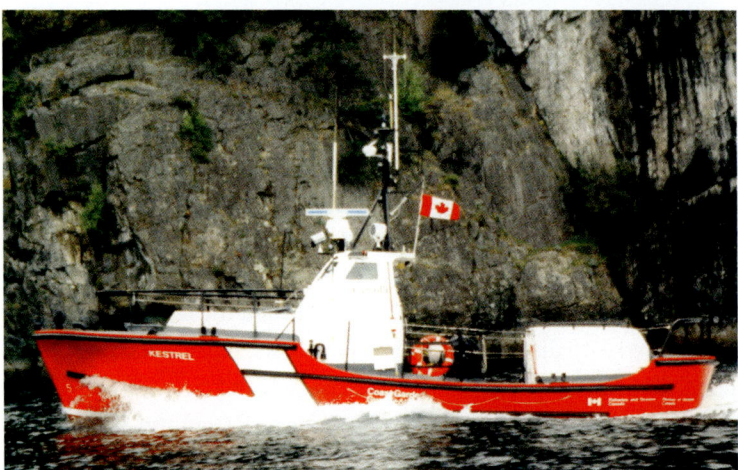

◢ Canadian Coast Guard 44ft Type 300 lifeboat CCGC Kestrel was built in 1969 at Chantier maritime de Saint-Laurent, Paspebiac, Quebec. She served originally at Bickerton, Nova Scotia, as CCGC Bickerton from 1969 to 1989, then, renamed CCGC Kestrel, as a college training vessel at Sydney, Nova Scotia until 1994. She was at French Creek, British Columbia, from 1994 to 2004.

the lifeboat service in Portugal. Both were built by the Navy Shipyard in Portugal: the first, completed in 1978, was named Sota-Patrão António Crista, and the second, completed in 1979, was named Patrão Joaquim Casaca. In 1975 ten 44ft boats were built for the Imperial Iranian Navy by Fairey Marine at Cowes under licence from the US Government. The Iranian Navy paid $56,400 to the USCG but further details of these boats, and what they were used for, is lacking.

44-footers at the limits

The strength and sturdiness of the 44ft lifeboat is perhaps best illustrated by the following statistics: by 1995 CG-44300 had capsized six times, pitchpoled end-over-end three times and once been rammed by a freighter. Yet it was still afloat and had kept its crews alive, proving that the 44-footer was able to cope in the most extreme circumstances. The ability to self-right, an essential requirement of the original design, was clearly necessary for operations in the heavy surf typically found on the US west coast. The huge breaking waves at the river bars are often over 20ft in height, and make the possibility of capsizing high. Indeed, the self-righting abilities of the design were put to the test soon after it entered service as, within five years of becoming operational, three had capsized and righted, without loss of life.

One of these capsizes occurred on the Umpqua River Bar, Oregon on 11 June 1966, when CG-44303 was on patrol, with CG-36514 standing by craft coming into the river through breaking swells 25ft in height and more. While guarding the danger areas, a series of large swells began moving in, picking up height as they approached CG-44303. CG-44303 was in a trough and running with the swell, but her bow was digging into the back of the swell ahead. As the seas astern broke, the stern of CG-44303 was caught in the curl of the wave and the boat was turned over. The Coxswain, Thomas McAdams, shouted 'hang on' to the other crew members just before all were submerged.

The boat settled in the overturned position and then slowly righted itself. The Coxswain was strapped into his seat and remained there; another crew member was thrown against the preventer screen at the rear of the wheelhouse; and the third crew member was washed overboard, but was soon picked up once the boat had righted. Both engines were still running, in neutral, after the capsize, and after the

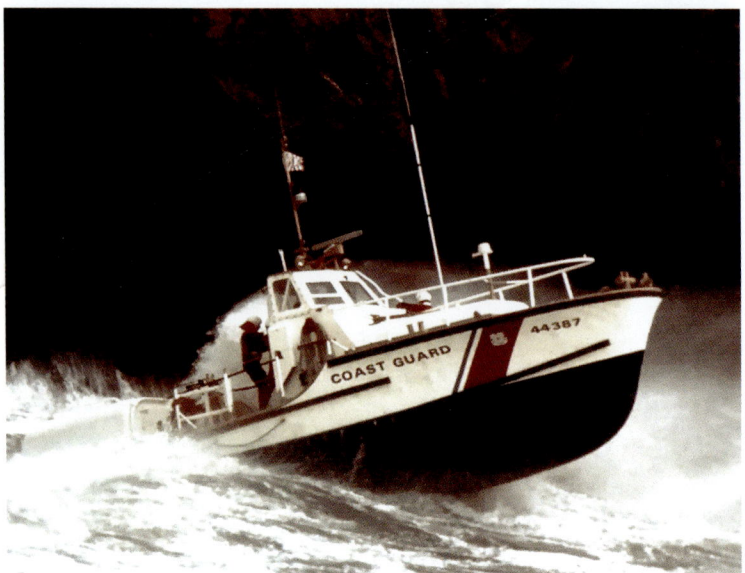

US Coast Guard 44ft motor lifeboat 44387 in surf conditions off Grays Harbor, on the coast of Washington, typical of the conditions encountered on the country's Pacific coast. (By courtesy of the USCG)

third crew member had been picked out of heavy swell the boat was taken into calm water where the crew examined her.

During the capsize approximately 1,000 gallons of water was sucked into the engine room and oil spilled from the hydraulic starting motor reservoir. Apart from this, much of the gear had survived, with most damage occurring on the topside of the vessel. Everything above the deckhouse had been carried away or been bent out of shape. The mainmast and radar scanner and the fire hose were gone. In his report of the incident, Coxswain McAdams noted that, while the 44-footer performed extremely competently in rough seas, being caught in the curl of a large breaker was the most dangerous position to be in, although the boat's inherent structural resilience ensured the boat and crew's survival.

As a result of this capsize, a study of the behaviour of equipment on board CG-44303 was undertaken by USCG design teams, who recommended a number of minor changes to the design. CG-44303 was delayed in righting when her superstructure struck the bottom. Tests on the righting behaviour showed that the boat would not right unless external forces rolled it forty degrees from the capsized vertical. To improve the boat's righting capabilities, the centre of buoyancy was raised, the centre of gravity lowered, and buoyant foam was placed on the underside of the wheelhouse roof. With regard to engine room flooding, which would also have a detrimental effect on the boat's righting ability, an automatic shut-off was fitted so that, if the boat was in the capsized position, the engines would not continue to run and suck water through the air intake ducts.

Since the first checks on the boat's self-righting ability were made in 1967, periodic assessments have taken place to monitor the boats' stability. In 1967 it was evident that, although the boat was stable in the capsized position, the forces needed to bring the boat upright were so small that alterations were unnecessary. Further tests were made in May 1971 when CG-44396 was capsized under controlled conditions at the Coast Guard Yard. Modifications made since 1967, such as the removal of both hydraulic starting systems and lower rubber fenders, reduced the boats' weight, and this had improved the righting capabilities.

The 44-footer's righting ability was put to the test again on 26 November 1973, when CG-44373 rolled over four times in heavy surf at Gleneden Beach, Oregon. All four crew members, having been thrown off the boat, were rescued from the water by helicopter. The most serious injury any of them sustained was a fractured shoulder blade. The boat lost its windshield structure, all exterior electronics, and the forward and after cabin tops as well as the engine vents were partially crushed. However, the engines were still running when the boat was washed up on the beach and only about 300 gallons of water had entered

▼ Three 44ft motor lifeboats rafted together, left to right: 44300 (Yaquina Bay), which capsized six times during her USCG career; 44381 from Mackinac Island; and 44369 from Neah Bay. (By courtesy of the USCG)

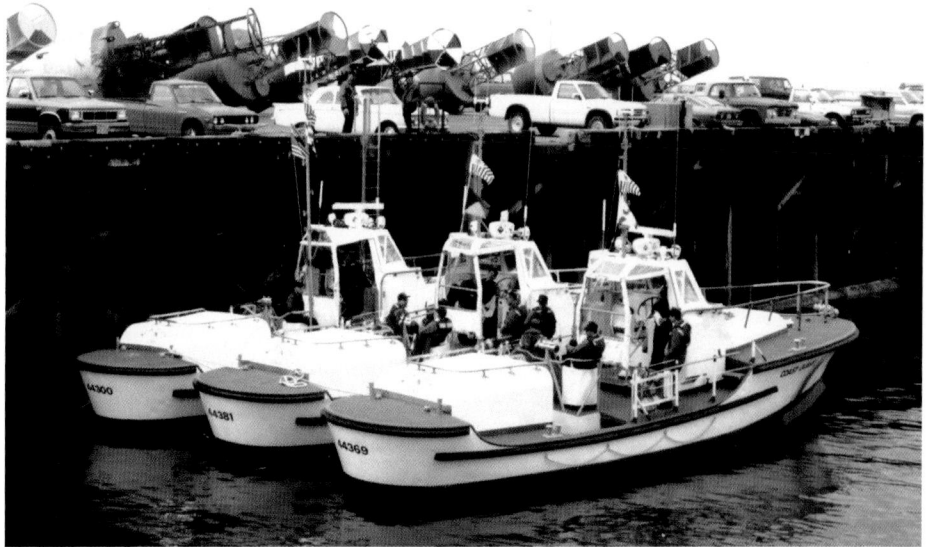

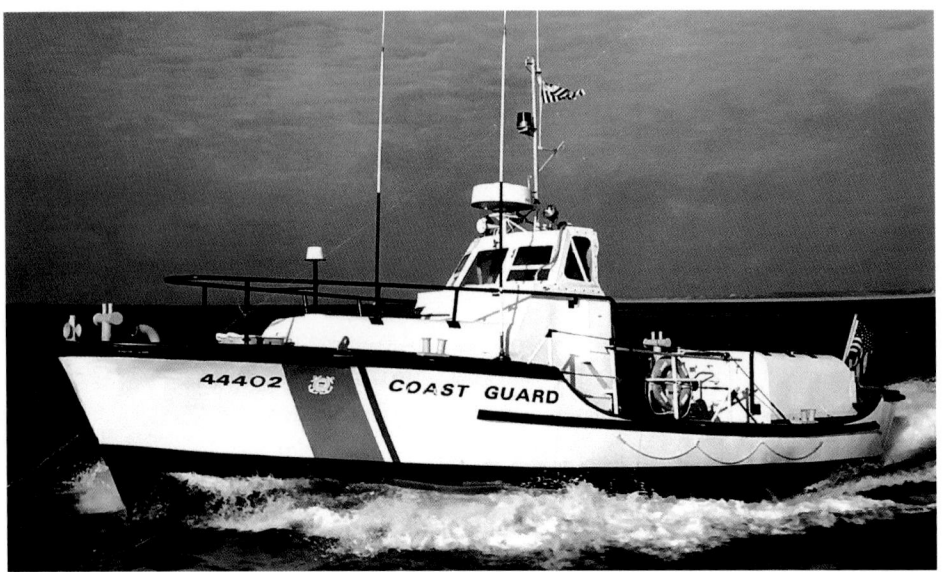

▲ US Coast Guard 44ft motor lifeboat 44402, one of the last ten 44-footers built for the USCG, served at USCG Station Chatham, Boston, Massachusetts. (By courtesy of the USCG)

the engine room. The boat grounded in the upright position and this, together with the fact that the engines were still running, was testament to the seaworthiness of the boat, the excellence of the original design, its strong construction and the high standards of maintenance.

Further capsizes of USCG 44ft motor lifeboats have occurred. In 1975 one capsized in Alaska and, although the crew were rescued, the boat itself was lost. Sadly, the crew of one of the two 44ft motor lifeboats from the Quillayute River Station were not so fortunate in February 1997, when their boat capsized. Of the four Coastguardsmen on board, three were lost: Seaman Clinton Miniken, Petty Officer Second Class David Bosley and Petty Officer Third Class Matthew Schlimme. Nineteen-year-old Seaman Apprentice Benjamin Wingo, the most junior member of the team, survived. This was the first capsizing of a 44-footer in thirty-five years of USCG service in which crews' lives had been lost.

The capsized boat was one of two sent out from the Quillayute River Station, along with a helicopter, to assist two people on a sailing vessel who radioed that they were taking on water in heavy seas. The 44-footer got caught parallel to incoming waves and, in the trough of two waves, capsized three times and was washed ashore inside a cove on James Island, just off the coast. Each time it capsized, it righted as designed, but the crew were washed overboard. District Commander for the Pacific

Northwest, Coast Guard Admiral J. David Spade, later commented: 'It's the worst tragedy I have ever experienced in my command'.

Capsized on service

The Waveneys built in Britain had aluminium, rather than steel, decks and wheelhouses. This reduced weight above the waterline, which in turn lowered the centre of gravity and improved the righting ability by making the boat less stable in the inverted position. Only one RNLI Waveney has capsized on service. On 28 February 1993 the Hartlepool lifeboat The Scout (44-018) was twice capsized in severe conditions off the north-east coast of England while she was on service to the tanker Freja Svea. The lifeboat was standing by the tanker when, climbing at an angle up a 30ft to 40ft sea, she was laid over hard to port as she neared the wave's curling crest. With no water on the other side, she fell into the trough of the wave and capsized.

The lifeboat performed exactly as designed and righted on both occasions, with none of the crew being lost, although some sustained minor injuries. One crew member, Robbie Maiden, was washed overboard, but was safely picked up by an RAF helicopter after spending thirty-five minutes in the water, having inflated his life-jacket. The lifeboat was damaged by the force of the water and escorted back to station by the lifeboat from the neighbouring Teesmouth station, the 47ft Tyne Phil Mead. Only minor structural damage was sustained. The mast had been sheared off, the searchlight was bent and the after

▼ The damage suffered by Hartlepool's Waveney The Scout (44-018) during the capsizes in February 1993 was mainly to the aerials and mast on the wheelhouse (right). The forward rope storage box (left) was bent by the force of water during the capsizes. (Supplied by R.W. Williams)

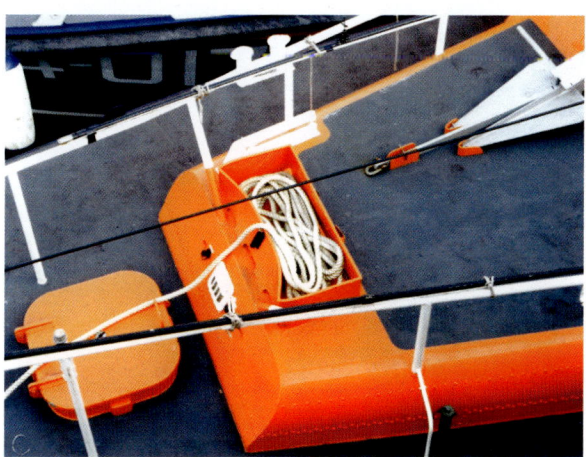

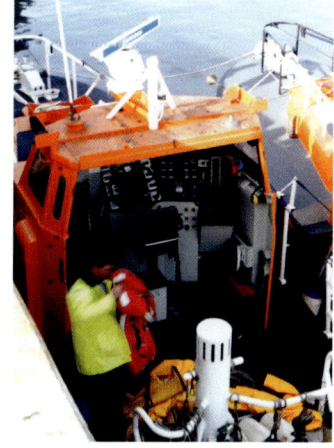

cabin had some indentations, and bolts holding down the Coxswain's seat were sheered off when a crew member was thrown against the seat, but the superstructure was intact and watertight and the boat was seaworthy. The RNLI's official report on the incident concluded: 'it is felt the lifeboat survived the service with flying colours'.

RNLI medal-winning services

Waveneys performed thousands of services around the coasts of Britain and Ireland, with a number of outstanding rescues undertaken in extreme conditions. The following accounts cover some of the more significant rescues undertaken in Waveneys, for which the RNLI awarded gallantry medals.

GREAT YARMOUTH & GORLESTON • November 1969 • On 9 November 1969 Khami (44-003) was launched in a westerly gale with very rough seas and heavy rain squalls to assist the Danish motor coaster Karen Bravo, which was in distress and listing heavily five miles south east of the Cross Sand lightvessel. In storm force ten conditions, with extremely rough confused seas, the lifeboat went alongside the casualty's starboard side seven times in order to take off five members of the crew. The lifeboat then escorted the vessel to Gorleston. In recognition of his courage, determination and superb seamanship, the Bronze Medal was awarded to Coxswain John Bryan.

▼ Khami on station at Great Yarmouth & Gorleston, where she served for almost thirteen years. She was involved in three Bronze medal-winning services during that time.

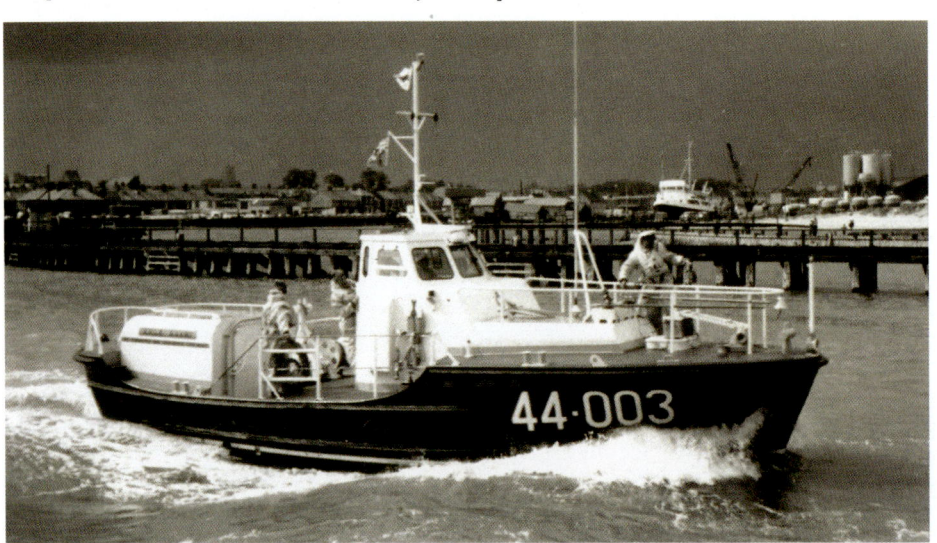

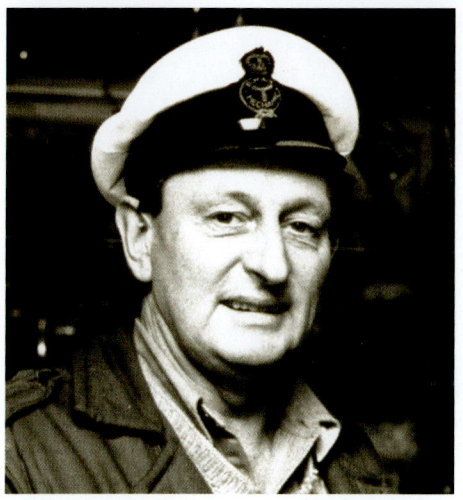
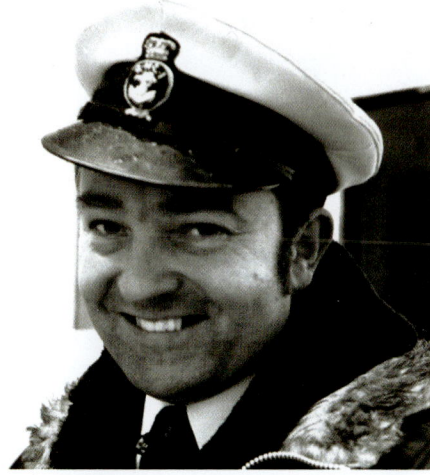

GREAT YARMOUTH & GORLESTON • December 1979 • On 22 December 1979 Khami (44-003) was launched to the fishing vessel St Margarite which was aground on the Scroby Sand, being washed by heavy breaking swell and sea. The wind was force six with a rough, steep sea, and approaching the casualty was difficult because the lifeboat was touching the bottom in the troughs. However, Khami was successfully taken alongside long enough for the two men on board to be rescued, although the lifeboat hit the bottom in the process. Once the two men were on board, the lifeboat pulled clear of the bank and stood by the abandoned vessel. When the fishing vessel bounced clear of the bank, at 7.15pm, the lifeboat crew rigged a tow line and towed the vessel back to Gorleston, although she later sank at her moorings. For this service, the Bronze medal was awarded to Coxswain Richard Hawkins, and medal service certificates were presented to the remainder of the crew, Second Coxswain Michael Brown, Stanley Woods, John Cooper and David Parr. The hull of Khami was undamaged during this service, despite the punishment it had taken on East Anglia's notorious sandbanks.

▲ Great Yarmouth & Gorleston medal recipients: John Bryan (left), Coxswain from 1967 to 1976, and his successor, Richard Hawkins, who served in the post for twenty years. Both were awarded Bronze medals for rescues undertaken in Khami, the first of two Waveneys built for service at Gorleston. (By courtesy of the RNLI)

SHEERNESS • March 1980 • On the night of 19 March 1980 Helen Turnbull (44-009) was launched to the Radio Caroline ship Mi Amigo, which was dragging her anchor in Black Deep near the Long Sand Bank, twenty-four miles from the station, in a severe gale force nine and very rough seas. While on passage to the casualty, the lifeboat had to reduce speed as she was shipping water and pounding heavily in the rough

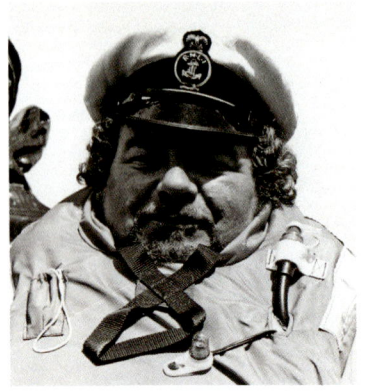

▲ Coxswain Charles Bowry of Sheerness, Silver and Bronze medal recipient for services aboard Helen Turnbull (44-009) in December 1978 and March 1980. (By courtesy of the RNLI)

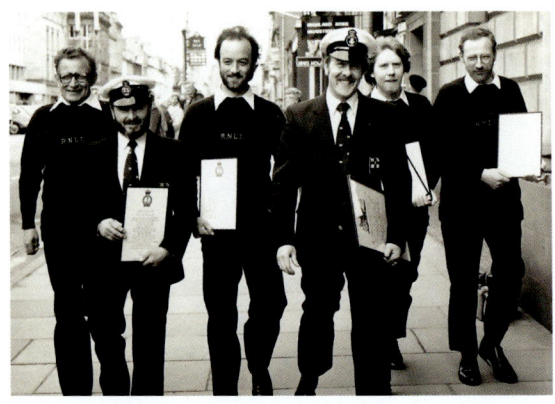

▲ The Troon lifeboat crew involved in the Silver medal service to the tug Holland I in Edinburgh for the Scottish Lifeboat Conference. Pictured are, left to right, Peter McClure, Tom Devenney (Second Coxswain), David Seaward, Ian Johnson (Coxswain), Roy Trewern, and Robert Hannah. (Courtesy of Ian Johnson)

seas. Once on scene, the lifeboat was manoeuvred alongside Mi Amigo in confused seas, facing an extreme rise and fall which made working in shallow water very hazardous. The lifeboat was brought alongside the casualty thirteen times, with many of the attempts being abandoned as the lifeboat was in danger of being stranded on the casualty's deck. During these many approaches, the four crew were taken off, one by one. On one approach, the lifeboat slammed against the side of the ship but luckily nobody was injured, and once the last of the crew had been taken off, the lifeboat headed into deeper water.

For this service, the Silver medal was awarded to Coxswain Charles Bowry; the Thanks inscribed on Vellum was accorded to the rest of the crew: Second Coxswain Arthur Lukey, Assistant Mechanic Roderick Underhill and crew Malcolm Keen, Ian McCourt and William Edwards.

TROON • September 1980 • On 12 September 1980 the Waveney stationed at Troon, on the Ayrshire coast of Scotland, Connel Elizabeth Cargill (44-007), was involved in an extremely challenging rescue. She was launched at 1.35pm under the command of Coxswain Ian Johnson in a a severe gale force nine gusting to force ten and very rough sea to the Dutch dredger Holland I. The dredger had been working off Irvine Harbour and was in danger of breaking her moorings in the strong winds. Waves up to 20ft high were sweeping across the dredger's main deck.

WAVENEY LIFEBOATS

The lifeboat cleared the harbour entrance and ploughed through confused seas for three miles to reach the casualty. Several times she was hit by huge waves that broke over her and at one point rolled so violently to starboard that the side of her wheelhouse was nearly in the water, but she reached the dredger at 2.20pm, finding her on the edge of the surf line with just a single stern mooring holding her. The lifeboat was taken alongside the casualty five times, with one man being taken off each time. On the first approach the lifeboat was thrown heavily against the dredger, damaging the Waveney's starboard plating. Each approach was very hazardous as the lifeboat would have been trapped by the dredger had the stern anchor cable broken.

The return passage to Troon was extremely difficult in the rough seas. Full power was required to drive her through the heavy seas off the harbour entrance but, once through, the survivors were safely landed ashore. For this rescue, the Silver medal was awarded to Coxswain Johnson in recognition of his courage, leadership and fine seamanship; medal service certificates were presented to the rest of the crew: Second Coxswain/Assistant Mechanic Thomas Devenny, Emergency Mechanics Peter McClure and David Seaward, and crew Robert Hannah and Roy Trewern.

RAMSGATE • December 1985 • Another Silver medal service involving a Waveney took place on 26 December 1985 when Ralph and Joy Swann (44-016), stationed at Ramsgate, went to the aid of the French trawler

▼ An oil painting by celebrated marine artist David Cobb showing Connel Elizabeth Cargill on service to the dredger Holland I in September 1980. The painting was displayed at the RNLI's headquarters in Poole. (By courtesy of the RNLI)

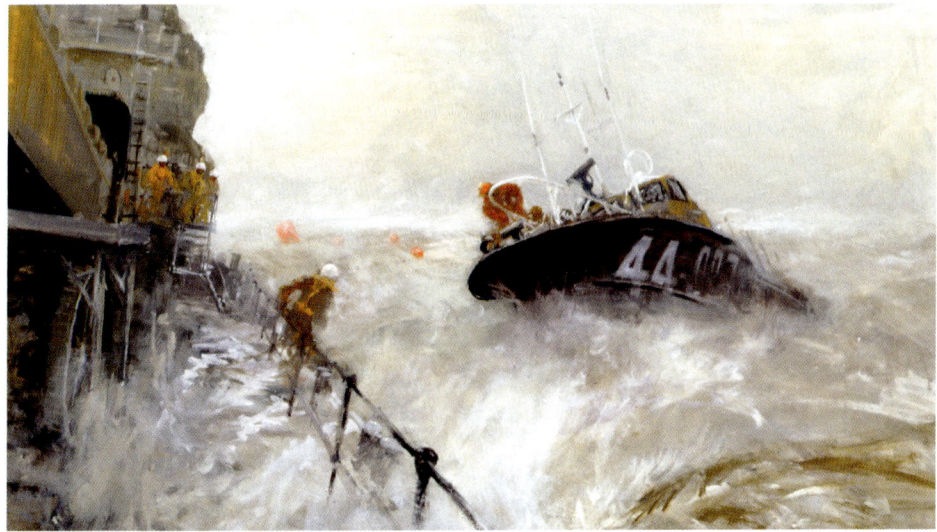

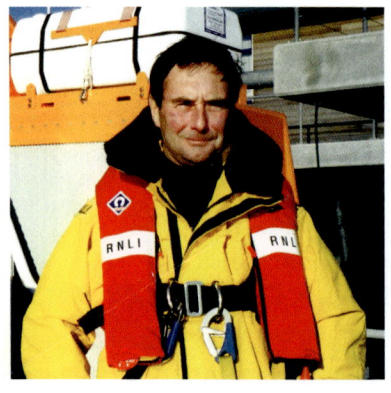

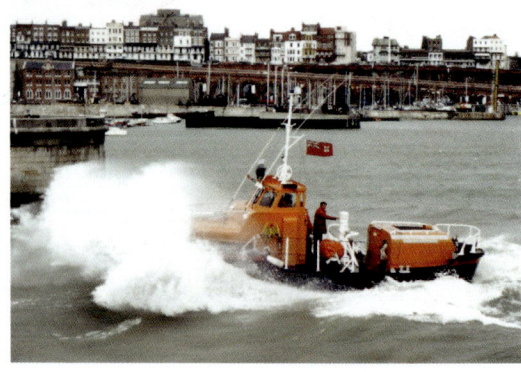

▲ Coxswain Ron Cannon served Ramsgate lifeboat for thirty-seven years, of which he was Coxswain for twenty-five. In the Waveney Ralph and Joy Swann (44-016) (pictured heading out of Ramsgate harbour), he received the Silver medal for saving a French trawler and its seven-man crew in 1985. (By courtesy of the RNLI; Ray Noble, right)

Gloire à Marie II, which was aground south of the port and in need of urgent assistance. The wind, already gale force nine, increased to a north-easterly violent storm force eleven. Because it was so rough in the harbour, Coxswain Ron Cannon and three crew used his father's 35ft workboat rather than the station's smaller boarding boat to board the lifeboat before bringing her alongside the pier to collect the remaining crew.

With waves reaching more than 30ft in height at the harbour entrance, Coxswain Cannon checked all the crew individually to make sure lifejackets and protective clothing were being properly worn before Ralph and Joy Swann headed to the harbour entrance at 8.15pm, being driven out into violent short cross seas. Once clear of the harbour, a course was set for the trawler with the lifeboat pitching and rolling heavily. At 10.25pm the casualty was seen aground in shoal water off the entrance to the river Stour. The irregular seas made the lifeboat difficult to control and a constant watch astern was maintained to warn of any steep seas. In order to help the casualty, two lifeboatmen were put on board, but getting the lifeboat alongside the trawler required considerable skill and several attempts had to be abandoned.

The skipper of the trawler did not want to abandon his vessel, particularly as it was seaworthy and the main engines were available. So Coxswain Cannon attempted to tow her off the sandbank on which she was stuck. A sixty-fathom towline was rigged, and then the lifeboat slowly began pulling the trawler's head round to the south, an extremely difficult manoeuvre which was skilfully executed. Twice, the heavy seas caused the towline to part, but it was reconnected. Once the trawler was clear of the sandbank, her engines were started and under her own power she was led to Ramsgate by Ralph and Joy Swann. Those in the harbour could not remember worse weather than on that night, when nine boats sank at their moorings inside the harbour. For this outstanding service, the Silver medal was awarded to Coxswain Cannon. Silver medal service certificates were presented to the remainder of the crew: Second Coxswain Derek Pegden, and crew Ronald Blay, Alan Bray, Michael Petts, Nigel Stephens, Ray Noble and John Cheeseman.

SHEERNESS • October 1987 • Another fine service using a Waveney was performed on 16 October 1987, when the crew of Helen Turnbull (44-009), at Sheerness, faced high winds and heavy seas as much of southern England was struck by a major hurricane, which caused severe damage both on land and at sea. Helen Turnbull put out at about 6am after red flares had been sighted. As the lifeboat headed out to sea, winds in excess of ninety knots were recorded, and at one point she was hit by an extremely heavy breaking sea, which swung her round so she was beam-on to the waves, but Coxswain Robin Castle, through skilful use of the engines, managed to bring the lifeboat round and back on course.

In waves up to 25ft high, the lifeboat was pitching and rolling violently, while visibility was reduced to almost zero by flying spray and the frequent heavy rain squalls. At 7.17am the casualty, a 16ft cabin cruiser,

▼ Helen Turnbull (44-009) heading out of Sheerness on 16 October 1987 at the height of the hurricane, since termed the 'Great Storm of 1987'. (By courtesy of the RNLI)

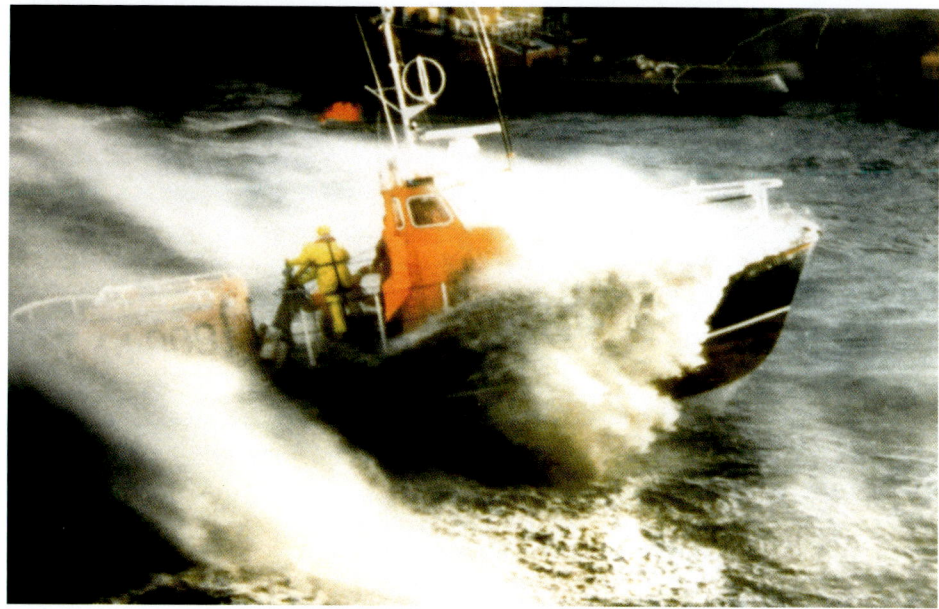

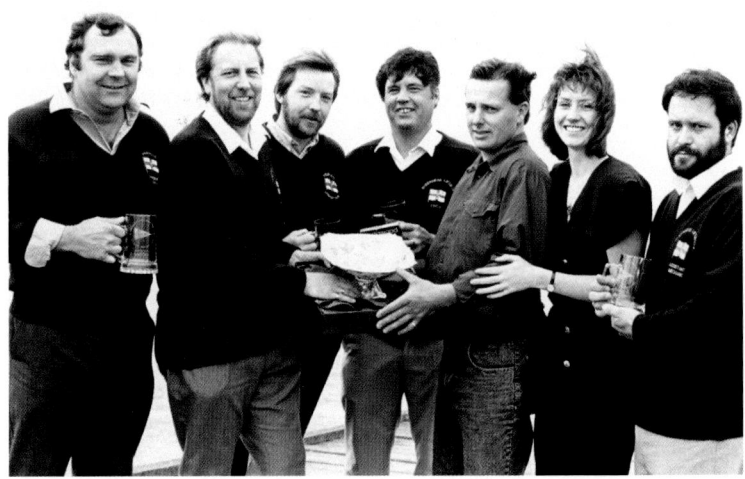

▶ Coxswain Robin Castle (second left) and the Sheerness crew being presented with a Crown Derby fruit bowl and engraved tankards for saving Tony Wells during the hurricane-force winds of October 1987. Tony and his wife also donated £230 for the station funds. (By courtesy of the RNLI)

was spotted by one of the lifeboatmen, and was seen to be slowly sinking as huge waves crashed over her. Despite the shallow water in which the casualty was stranded, Coxswain Castle took the lifeboat alongside and the two men on board were quickly hauled aboard the lifeboat. As Coxswain Castle came astern to clear the cruiser, a gust of wind swung the lifeboat around, her stern ran aground and, despite strenuous efforts on the part of the lifeboatmen, she remained fast.

After assessing the situation, the engines were shut down and the lifeboatmen, except the Coxswain and Second Coxswain, went below deck and the watertight doors were closed, with the VHF radio left on to maintain contact with the shore. When the water receded, the lifeboat crew examined the lifeboat's hull to ensure no damage had been sustained. Both propellers and rudders were found to be clear and, with the tide rising, the lifeboat floated clear. Using the spare anchor she was hauled off the sands and headed back to Sheerness Docks.

For this service, the Bronze medal was awarded to Coxswain Castle for his truly outstanding seamanship. The Thanks inscribed on Vellum was accorded to Second Coxswain Dennis Bailey and lifeboatman Richard Rogers, while Medal Service Certificates were presented to the rest of the crew, Peter Bullin, Eamon Finch and Brian Spoor. These services were carried out in extreme conditions and proved the exceptional design and construction of the 44ft Waveneys, with their sturdiness and power enabling the saving lives on many occasions.

Waveneys after service

At the start of the twenty-first century none of the RNLI's Waveneys remained in service. Their withdrawal and replacement began in the mid-1990s and, over the course of about four years starting in late 1996, all twenty-two boats were replaced on operational duty and sold out of service. The majority of the boats were sold abroad for further service as rescue craft, with six boats going to the Royal Volunteer Coastal Patrol in Australia and a further six being sold to Volunteer Coastguard units in New Zealand. Three of the boats became pilot boats, at Montrose, Berwick and Whitby, while only two entered private ownership in the UK, one of which was used for fishing charters and the other as a pleasure boat. Sea rescue organisations in Canada, Namibia and Uruguay each took one Waveney which continued serving as a lifeboat, while one sold into private ownership was taken as far as the Falkland Islands, where she remains.

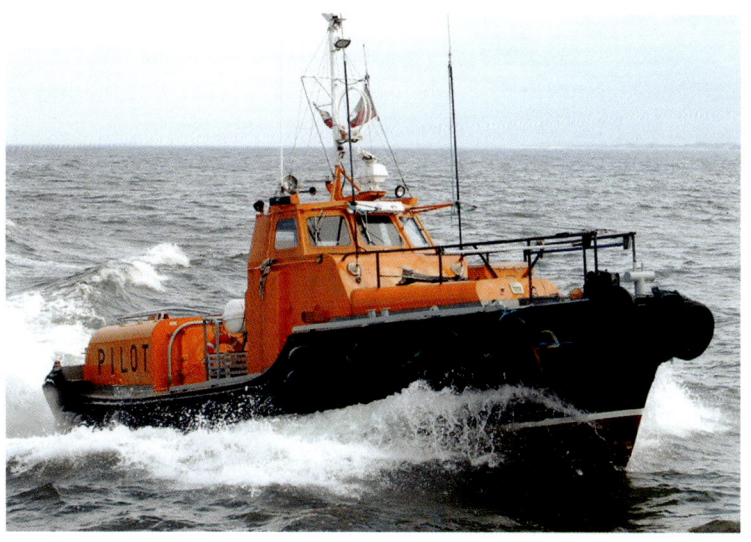

◀ The first Waveney to be sold out of service was Lady of Lancashire (44-015), which was bought by Berwick Harbour Commissioners in November 1996 and has, since then, served as the pilot vessel St Boisil. (Cliff Crone)

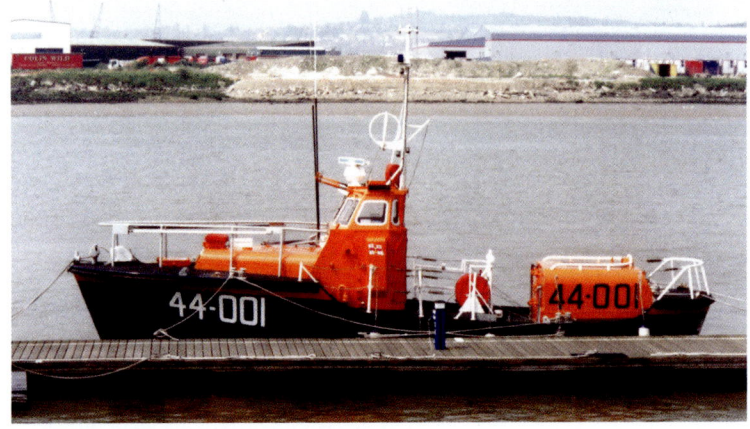

▶ The prototype Waveney 44-001 at moorings alongside Thunderbolt Pier, Chatham Dockyard in the River Medway. She was subsequently taken out of the water for static display ashore. She is one of the most important lifeboats of the twentieth century and her preservation ensures that the significance of the 44ft design will not be forgotten.

Prototypes on display

What became of the prototype 44-footer CG-44300 and her UK counterpart 44-001? Fortunately for those concerned with the history of lifesaving, both craft have been preserved and are displayed in the countries where they served. CG-44300 was handed over to the Columbia River Maritime Museum having been withdrawn from service after experiencing a serious engine breakdown during a search and rescue mission off Cape Disappointment on 29 July 1996. Although the boat was in good condition, the cost of repairing the damaged engine could not be justified, particularly as the 44-footers were being replaced by new 47ft motor lifeboats.

So, after a survey, CG-44300 was handed over to the Columbia River Maritime Museum in 1998, where she joined the collection of historic vessels. With her equipment and accessories intact, bearing the scars of her long career with the USCG, she is displayed at the Museum as the centrepiece of the story of the men and women of the US Coast Guard. The display focuses on the rescues on the Columbia River bar and how the USCG has helped to make the Columbia River safer.

Meanwhile the British prototype, 44-001, went to Chatham Historic Dockyard in 1997 to form part of the National Lifeboat Collection. For three years she was moored on the Medway at Thunderbolt Pier, which is part of the Historic Dockyard, and in June 1999 was taken to Poole by a team of museum volunteers to participate in the celebrations and parade of sail to mark the RNLI's 175th Anniversary.

Waveneys go 'down under'

In May 1999 the Royal Volunteer Coastal Patrol (RVCP) of Australia agreed to purchase six Waveneys, which had recently been taken out of RNLI service and were readily available in operational conditions. The RVCP, established in 1937 as Australia's first volunteer marine rescue organisation, operates around twenty-five bases, from Eden to Byron Bay. During the 1990s the rescue craft available for service in Australia were deemed unsuitable, and the Waveneys were regarded as a good

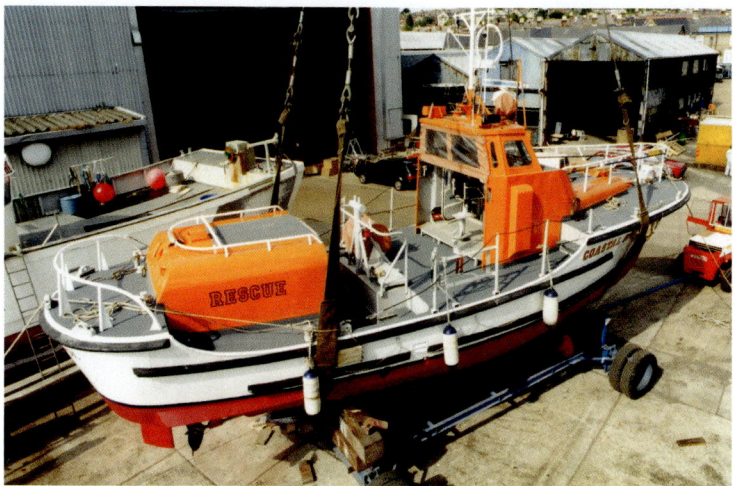

◀ 44-004 at Souter Shipyard, Cowes, being repainted for service with the RVCP in Australia, April 1999. (Peter Edey)

▼ 44-011 renamed P&O Nedlloyd Strathaird at Trial Bay, the station she served until 2011. (By courtesy of the RNLI)

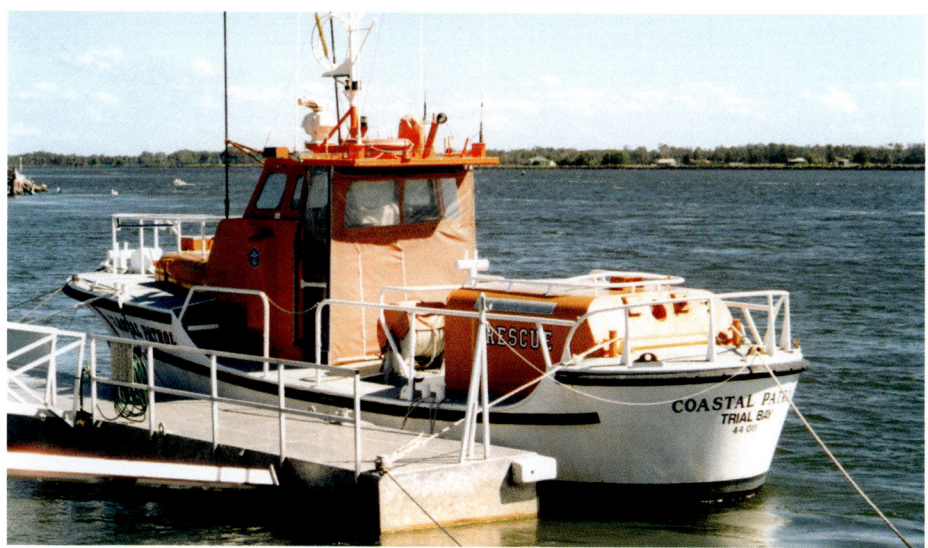

option. Of the six boats which went 'down under', four were part of the original half dozen built by Brooke Marine at Lowestoft.

Prior to going to Australia, the boats were taken to Souter Shipyard at Cowes, Isle of Wight, where they were repainted in the RVCP livery, being given white hulls. They were then shipped out as deck cargo on board P&O Nedlloyd container ships. Each boat was then renamed after the ship on which she had been transported to her new home: Strathmore (Narooma), Strathallan (Ulladulla/Broken Bay), Strathnaver (Batemans Bay), Stratheden (Botany Bay), Rawalpindi (Sydney/Port Jackson) and Strathaird (Trial Bay). The boats proved to be ideal, and were popular with their new crews. However, they were found to be very costly to maintain and were soon showing their age. After giving roughly a decade of service with the RVCP, they were sold into private hands.

Waveneys in New Zealand

As well as the six Waveneys which went to Australia, a further six were sold to New Zealand. The first sale was agreed in 1997, when the Royal New Zealand Coastguard Federation (RNZCF) decided to purchase Waveneys being offered for sale by the RNLI. Harold Mason, RNZCF National President, and his colleague, Lew Robinson, considered where the vessels would best be stationed in the country, and then negotiated a bulk purchase of Waveneys over three years.

The project was financed in part by the country's Lottery Grants Board, without whose help it would not have been possible. The RNLI covered the costs of getting the boats to Tilbury as well as loading charges at

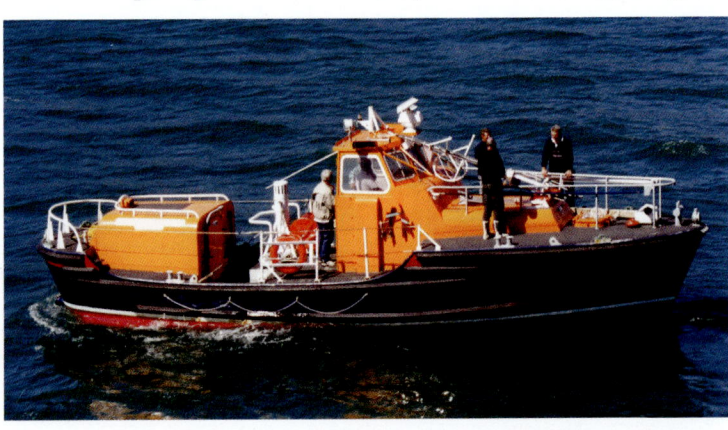

▶ 44-020 arriving in Wellington, New Zealand, on 22 October 1999, prior to entering service with Raglan Volunteer Coastguard. (By courtesy of V.H. Young)

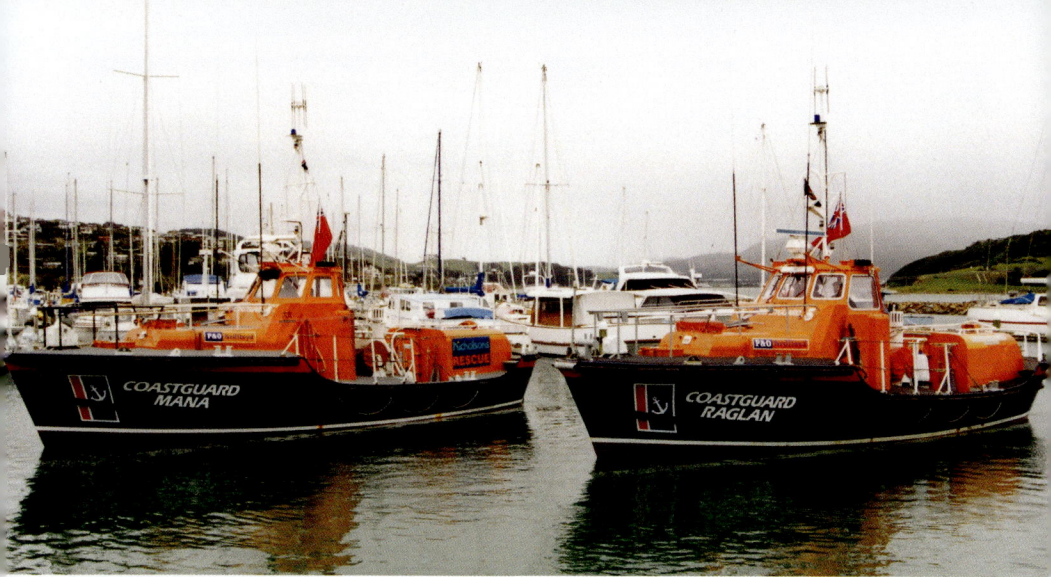

the port. P&O Nedlloyd agreed to ship the vessels free of charge, a sponsorship worth NZ$400,000. They had already shipped the RNLI's 33ft Brede lifeboat Amateur Swimming Associations (ON.1105) to New Zealand for service with the Nelson Volunteer Coastguard. In addition to the P&O Nedlloyd sponsorship, Port Wellington and Port Auckland container terminals provided unloading in New Zealand free of charge.

The first Waveney to arrive, Wavy Line (44-017), was allocated to Mana Volunteer Coastguard. She was brought to New Zealand on board the container ship Pegasus Bay and was renamed Nicholsons Rescue at a commissioning ceremony on 21 May 1998. The second, Louis Marchesi of Round Table (44-019), reached New Zealand on 4 April 1999 and was allocated to Waiheke Volunteer Coastguard. In 1999 David Acland, a Vice President of the RNLI, agreed to sponsor the Waveney for Kaikoura Volunteer Coastguard, The William and Jane (44-022), in memory of his great-great uncle John Barton Acland, who came to New Zealand 130 years previously, and so the boat was renamed John Barton Acland Rescue.

Kaikoura Coastguard (KCG) lobbied to have a Waveney assigned to the area, on the east coast of the south island of New Zealand, half way between Cook Strait and Banks Peninsula. Once allocated to KCG, 44-022 left Tilbury Docks on 30 May 1999, together with a Waveney destined for Australia, as deck cargo on board the container ship P&O Nedlloyd Palliser Bay. She arrived in Wellington, New Zealand, on 16 July

▲ 44-017 (on left), renamed Nicholsons Rescue, and 44-020, renamed Hamilton Rotary Rescue, entering service with New Zealand Coastguard. (By courtesy of V.H. Young)

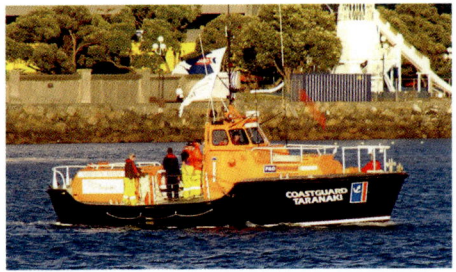
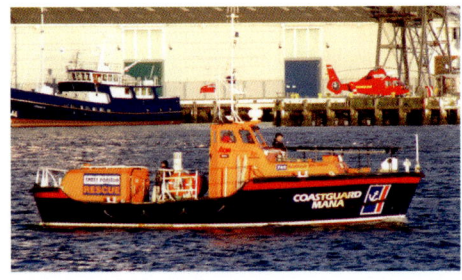

▲ 44-010 (left) was renamed Westgate Rescue and served Taranaki Coastguard in New Zealand from 1999 to 2012; 44-017 (right) served as Nicholsons Rescue with Mana Coastguard, near Wellington, from 1998 to 2010. (Supplied by Martin Fish)

1999 to be unloaded, free of charge, by the Wellington Port Company. The KCG crew prepared her for the passage to Kaikoura the following day, which involved crossing the notorious Cook Strait. The lifeboat arrived at Kaikoura at 4.30pm on Saturday 17 July 1999 after a relatively uneventful passage. She was subsequently slipped, anti-fouled, and had GPS and other equipment fitted before becoming operational. A berth was provided in the local Marina free of charge, and the formalities of the KCG's new acquisition were completed with both a church and Maori blessing on 20 November 1999.

Most of the Waveneys in New Zealand spent less than ten years in Coastguard service, before being sold into private hands. As with the Australian boats, they were found to be too slow, despite having good towing capabilities and being sufficiently rugged to face the worst conditions. A number of other Waveneys went abroad for continued lifesaving service: 44-012 served in Canada, 44-008 was acquired by the Sea Rescue Institute of Namibia, and 44-018 went to the Uruguayan lifeboat service ADES. None remain as rescue boats, apart from 44-008.

▶ 44-012 at Delta Station, Roberts Bank, Vancouver, Canada, where she served from 1999 to 2008. She was operated by the Canadian Lifeboat Institution, from 2002 by the Canadian Coast Guard Auxiliary and later by the Roberts Bank Lifeboat Society. (Supplied by Martin Fish)

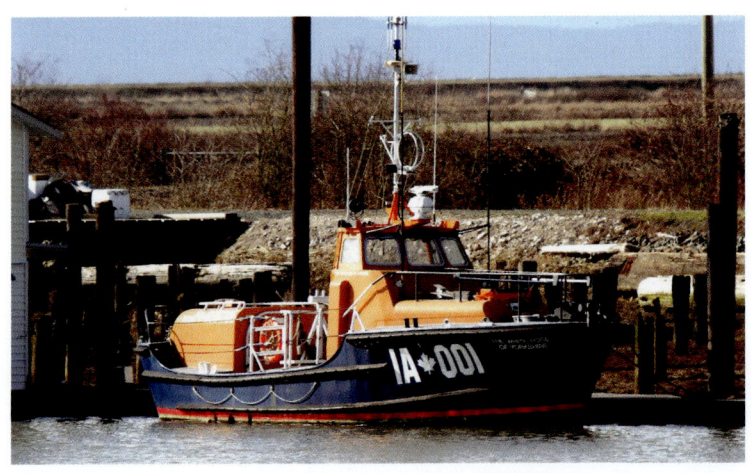

WAVENEY LIFEBOATS

Careers of the Waveneys

The RNLI built twenty-one 44ft Waveney lifeboats and, with the USCG-built boat 44-001, operated a fleet of twenty-two of the craft during the late 1960s and throughout the 1970s and 1980s, into the 1990s. The first British-built Waveney entered service at Dun Laoghaire in May 1967, the first of five Waveneys to become operational that year. The last Waveney to be built, 44-022, entered service at Blyth in October 1982. The last of the class in RNLI service, 44-005, was replaced at Amble in Northumberland in July 1999. None of the Waveneys were built specifically for the Relief Fleet, but many of the boats served in the Relief Fleet after they had been replaced at their original stations. Several of the first batch of six Waveneys enjoyed careers lasting almost three decades, and most of the rest gave at least two decades of service. The boats were well liked by the volunteer crews and thousands of rescues were carried out by the Waveneys.

▼ The William and Jane (44-022) was the last RNLI Waveney in operational service in Ireland when she was replaced at Larne by the 52ft Arun in November 1998. (By courtesy of the RNLI)

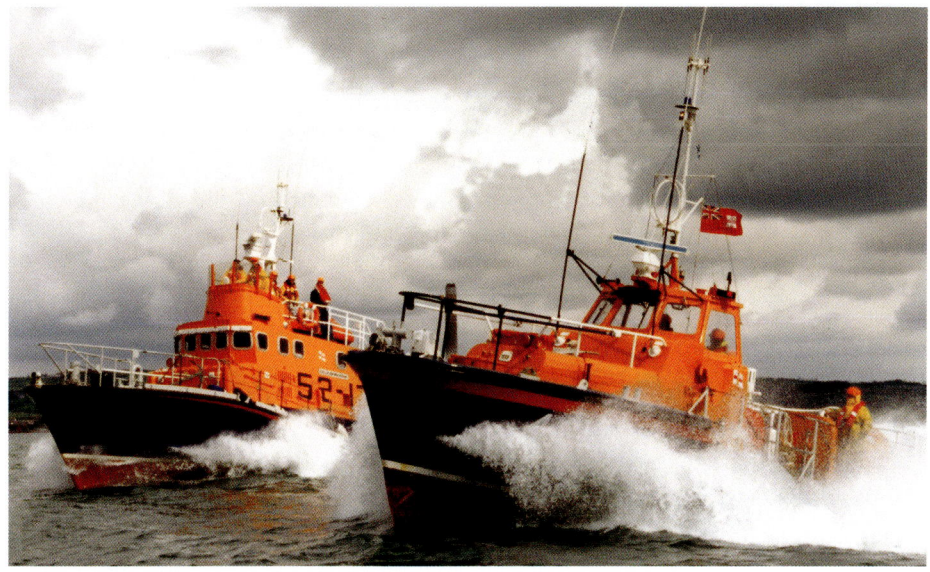

44-001

Key data

Built 1964, US Coast Guard Yard
Donor RNLI general funds
Stations Trials 1964 - 1967 (7/9), Relief Feb 1967 – Mar 1997 (291/100)
Disposal Displayed at Historic Lifeboat Collection, Chatham, from 1997

Service career

44-001, the prototype Waveney, was operated as a relief lifeboat for more then three decades and performed many rescues around the UK and Ireland. Probably the most outstanding took place on 6 October 1990 when she was at Eyemouth. In hurricane-force winds gusting to 100mph, accompanied by heavy rain with waves 20ft high at the harbour entrance, several divers needed help. With telephone lines down and maroons inaudible in the storm, neither Coxswain nor Second Coxswain could be contacted, so Assistant Mechanic James Dougal took command as Acting Coxswain and 44-001 headed out to sea through the appalling conditions at the harbour entrance. A course was set for St Abbs, where the divers had been reported, but speed had to be reduced as 35ft seas were encountered. 44-001, together with Dunbar lifeboat, searched for the divers, all crew on deck being secured by lifelines. At 5.20pm two divers were spotted just north of Ebb Carr Rocks, and they were pulled aboard the lifeboat. The two divers were suffering from severe seasickness, but conditions at St Abbs harbour were too severe to safely get the lifeboat through the narrow entrance. Both lifeboats made for Burnmouth but, as the harbour lights were out, a local fisherman, J. Johnston, arranged for two cars to be positioned to indicate the correct course with their headlights, to enable the lifeboats to enter the harbour. Both boats safely negotiated the entrance to Burnmouth Harbour. For this outstanding service, Acting Coxswain Dougal was awarded the Silver medal for taking the lifeboat to sea even though, due to the appalling conditions, Eyemouth was closed; the Thanks Inscribed on Vellum was accorded to the other crew members. Despite being more than 20 years old when this service took place, 44-001 performed superbly throughout and ensured a successful outcome.

After service

44-001 was withdrawn from service on 9 January 1996. In March 1997 she became part of the Historic Lifeboat Collection, at Chatham Dockyard, being used as a floating exhibit and to support local fundraising events, notably at Kingston upon Thames, Ramsgate and Whitstable. In May 2000 she was on display at Chatham Navy Days, her last official engagement before being lifted out of the water to become a static exhibition at Chatham's No.4 slipway.

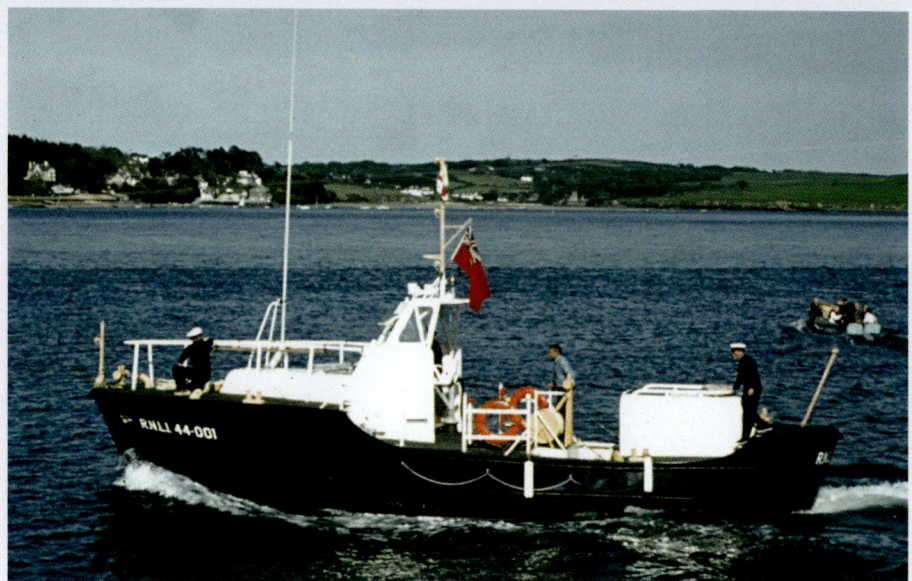

▲ 44-001 visiting Padstow during her tour around the British Isles, May 1964. (By courtesy of the RNLI)

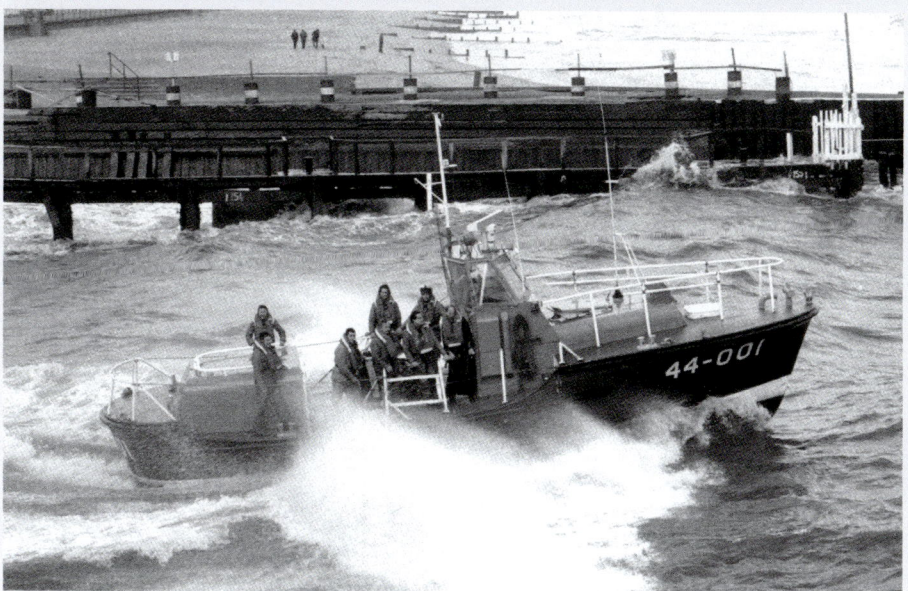

▲ 44-001 heading out of Gorleston harbour while on relief duty at the Norfolk station.

44-001

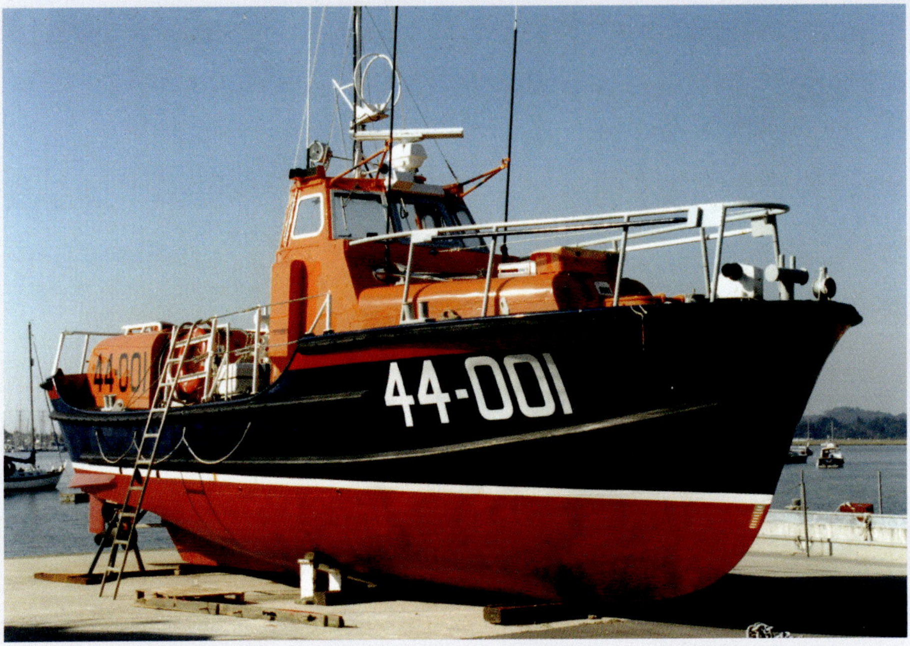

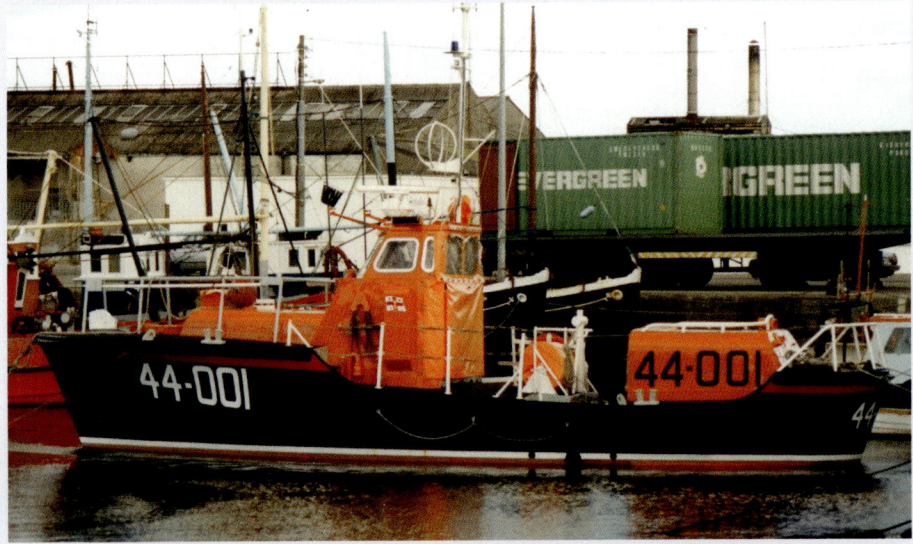

▲ 44-001 at the RNLI Depot, Poole, October 1994, thirty years after arriving in Britain. (Nicholas Leach)

▲ 44-001 on relief duty at Arklow, September 1995, during a three-month stint at the Irish station.

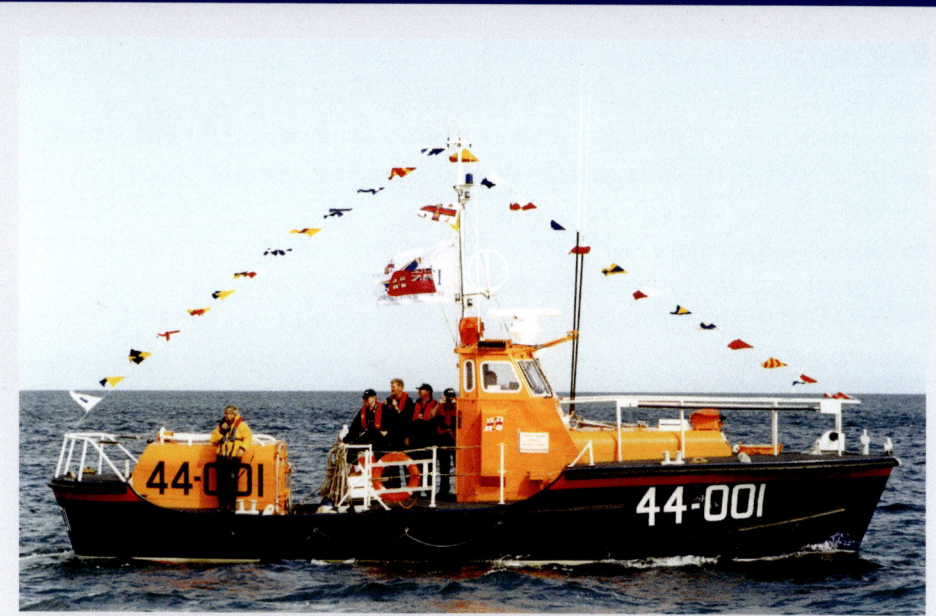

▲ 44-001 participating in the RNLI's 175th anniversary celebrations at Poole, with historic and international lifeboats, June 1999; she was manned by a group of volunteers from Chatham Dockyard. (Nicholas Leach)

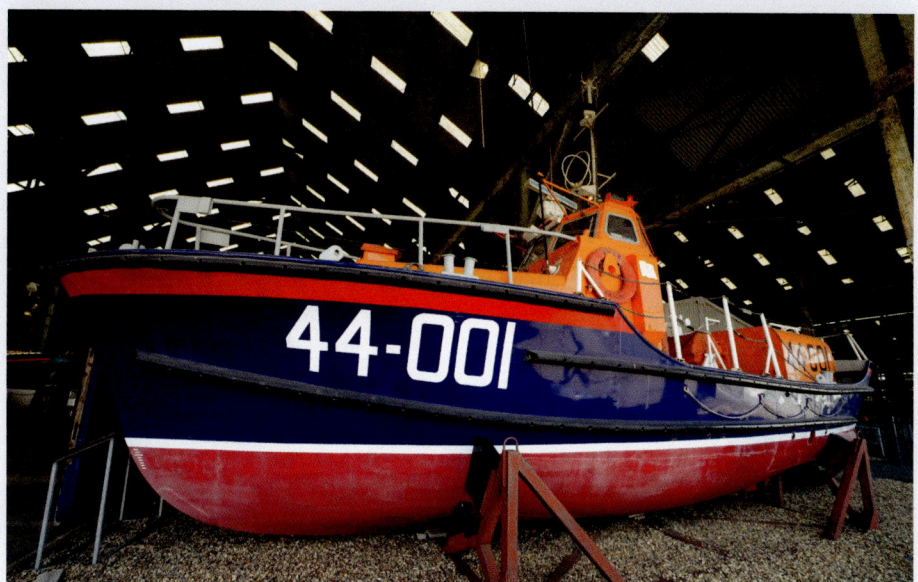

▲ 44-001 on display at the Lifeboat Collection, Chatham Historic Dockyard, May 2021. (Nicholas Leach)

John F. Kennedy

Key data

Built 1966, Brooke Marine, Lowestoft; yard no. B348
Donor Legacy of Miss Charlotte M.H. Gibson, Wellington, Somerset, and RNLI General Funds
Named 12 Aug 1967 at Dun Laoghaire by Mrs de Courcy Ireland, wife of the station's
    Honorary Secretary, John de Courcy Ireland
Stations Dun Laoghaire May 1967 – Apr 1990 (238/161), Relief Apr 1990 – 1996 (72/10)
Disposal Sold Aug 1996 to Alan Skinner, Newcastle-upon-Tyne

Service career

John F. Kennedy served at Dun Laoghaire for twenty-three years, covering the busy waters of Dublin Bay, after which she spent a further six years in the Relief Fleet. One of her more notable services was undertaken on 14 October 1980, when she went to help an injured seaman on the Norwegian bulk carrier Blix. The honorary medical advisor, Dr Niall Webb, was taken on board as John F. Kennedy put out and headed for the rendezvous position four miles east of Dun Laoghaire, reaching Blix just before 2am on 15 October. Getting the lifeboat alongside proved very difficult in the heavy swell, and Dr Webb had to jump from the lifeboat's bow onto the bulker's pilot ladder. The injured seaman, suffering from a fractured leg and rib, was then secured in a Neil Robertson stretcher to be transferred to the lifeboat. It took several attempts to take off the doctor, who had to jump onto the lifeboat on the instruction of the Second Coxswain. For this rescue, a special doctor's vellum was presented to Dr Webb, and a collective Letter of Appreciation signed by the RNLI Director, Rear Admiral W.J. Graham, was sent to Coxswain/Mechanic Eric Offer and his crew for their part in this service.

After service

John F. Kennedy was placed on the sale list on 22 August 1996 and sold out of service in August 1996 to Alan Skinner. Initially she was kept at Davy Bank, Newcastle, and her aft cabin was removed to make a larger working area aft, while the wheelhouse was enlarged and enclosed. Renamed Sarah JFK, she was licensed to carry twelve passengers on sea angling trips, and operated out of North Shields Fish Quay and Mill Dam, South Shields, on the river Tyne, later moving to a berth in Royal Quays Marina. In 2016 she was sold to Dave Burton of Bay Charters, Eastbourne and sailed to Eastbourne in April 2016, to be used as a charter boat, being renamed Fortitude. She was sold again in March 2018 and taken to Brixham, Devon. In September 2019 she was sold again, and was stripped out, being taken on low loader to the Thames and reportedly transported to Lagos, Nigeria.

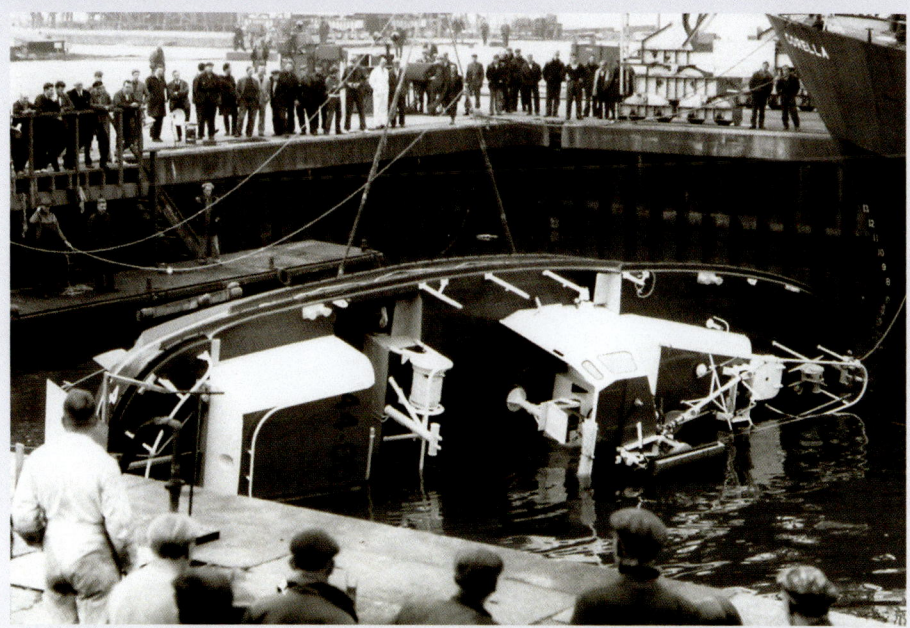

▲ 44-002 being tipped over as part of her capsize trials at Lowestoft. (By courtesy of the RNLI)

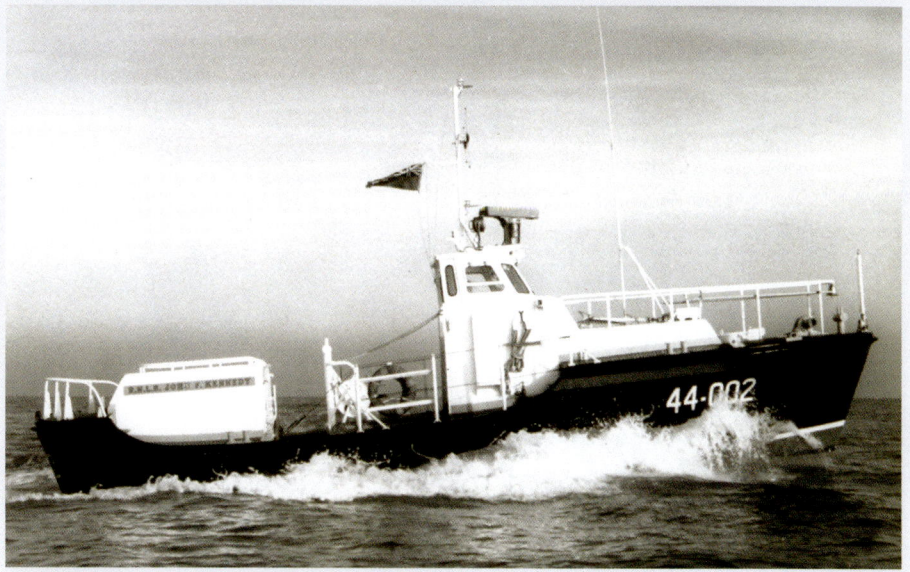

▲ 44-002 on exercise in Dublin Bay while she was on station at Dun Laoghaire.

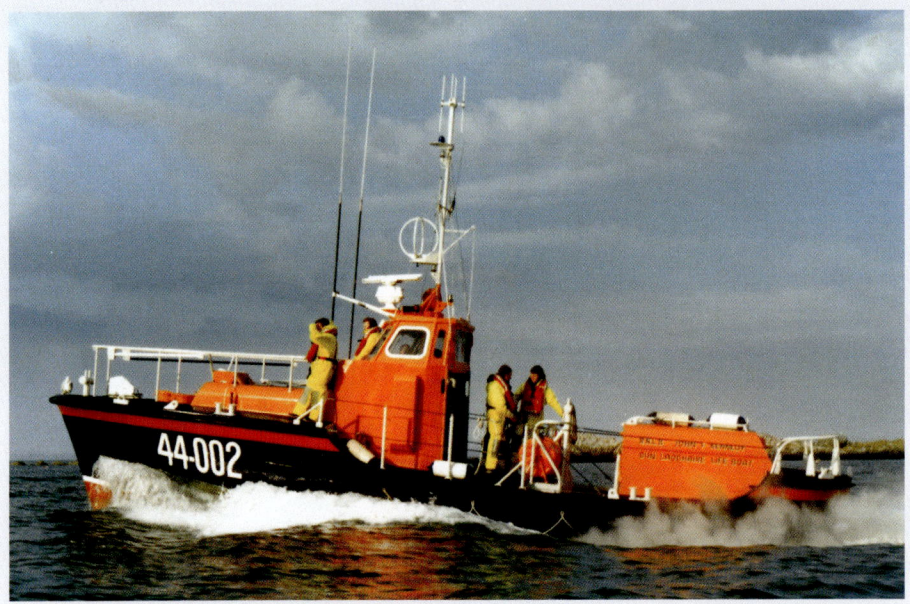

▲ 44-002 on exercise in Dublin Bay while she was on station at Dun Laoghaire.

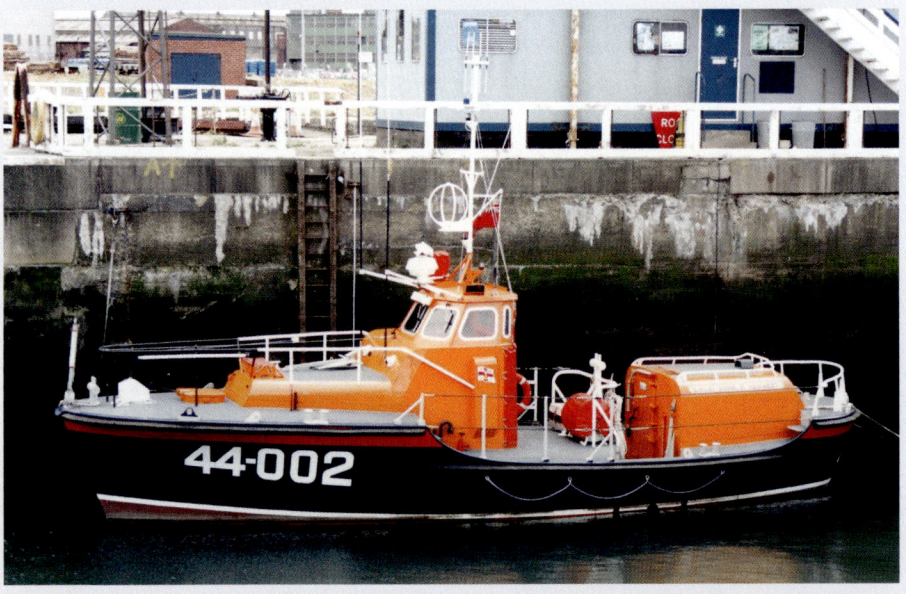

▲ 44-002 on relief at Hartlepool, where she spent two months on duty, August 1994. (Nicholas Leach)

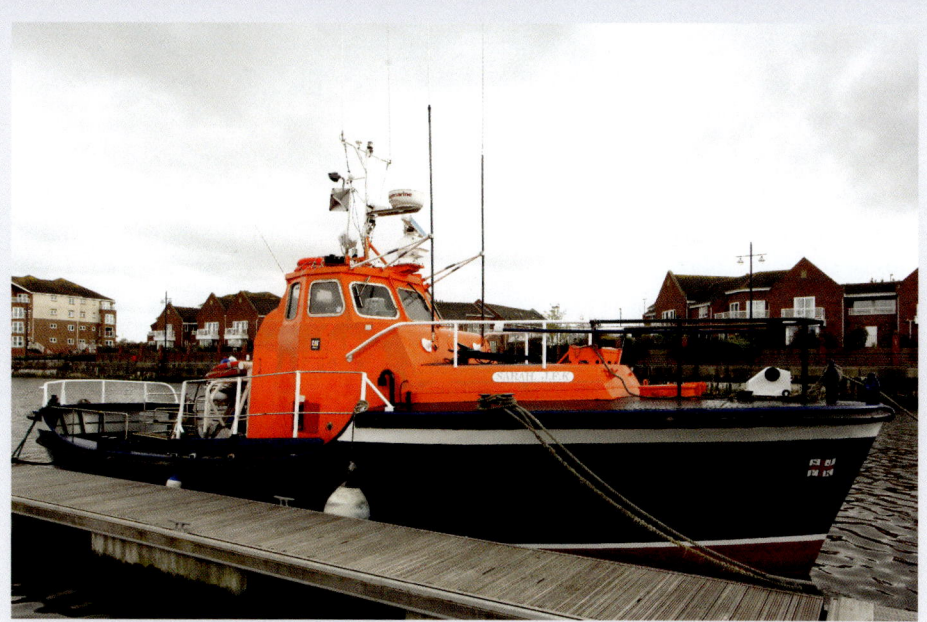

▲ 44-002 renamed Sarah JFK at Royal Quays Marina, Newcastle, April 2013. (Nicholas Leach)

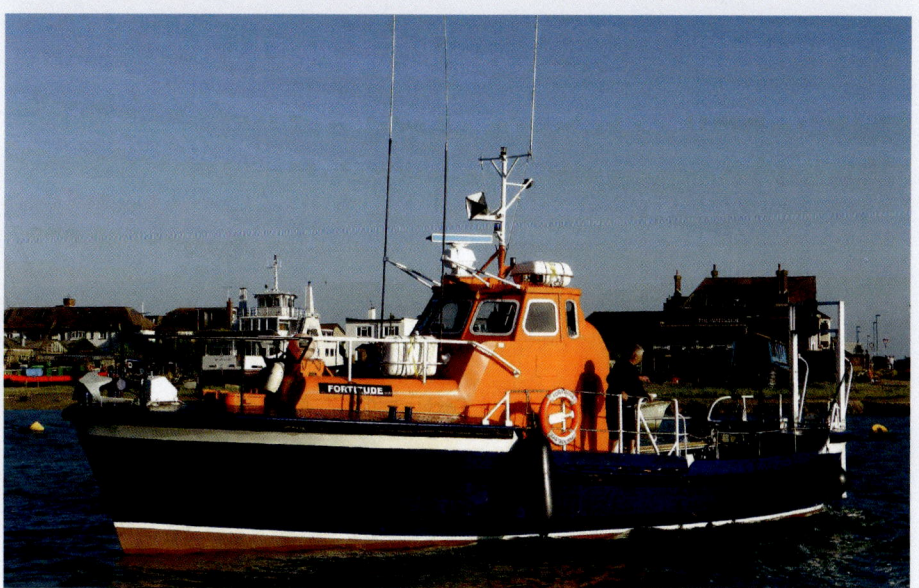

▲ 44-002 renamed Fortitude at Sussex Yacht Club, Shoreham, August 2016. (Philip Simons)

Key data

Built 1967, Brooke Marine, Lowestoft; yard no. B349

Donor Gift of Mr and Mrs T. G. Bedwell

Named 17 May 1967 at Gorleston-on-Sea by Mrs Bedwell after a settlement in Rhodesia where the donors once lived

Stations Great Yarmouth & Gorleston 19 Aug 1967 – May 1980 (234/71), Relief May 1980 – 1997 (240/90)

Disposal Placed on sale list on 11 May 1997, sold 21 May 1999 to RVCP, Australia

Service career

Khami served for the first thirteen years of her career at Great Yarmouth and Gorleston, where she was kept in a purpose-built pen on the west side of the River Yare. Among several notable rescues she performed while at Gorleston was that undertaken in the early hours of 13 December 1974 to the 493-ton motor vessel Biscaya, which had been in collision with a French tug. Under the command of Coxswain John Bryan, the lifeboat battled through a force nine gale to reach the vessel, which was forty-five miles south-east of Gorleston. She arrived on the scene at 6.30am and found the ship listing slightly with her steering gear out of action. The lifeboat stood by to await a tug, which arrived at 10.34am, by which time the casualty had begun to list severely. Three of her crew took to a liferaft and were picked up immediately by the lifeboat. The other three crew remained on board until 11.25am when the list increased. Coxswain Bryan then took the lifeboat close in and recovered the three men despite the heavy swell and the list making the transfer very difficult. For this service the Bronze second service clasp was awarded to Coxswain Bryan and medal service certificates to the rest of the crew. Following her time at Gorleston, Khami spent seventeen years in the Relief Fleet.

After service

Khami was sold on 21 May 1999 to the Royal Volunteer Coastal Patrol, Australia, for service in the Botany Bay Division, New South Wales, as a Coast Guard vessel and lifeboat. She was repainted in the livery of the Coastal Patrol (white hull) at Souter Shipyard, Cowes and kept at the RNLI Depot, Poole, until being shipped out to Australia. She was renamed P&O Nedlloyd Stratheden. In 2012 she was sold to a private buyer in Queensland, who resold her and in 2013 she was taken to Esperance, Western Australia. In July 2014 she was bought by Rowlie Walker, who sailed her from Esperance to Tamar River, Tasmania, covering 1,400 miles in eight days. She remains unaltered and used as a yacht club safety vessel at Launceston, Tasmania.

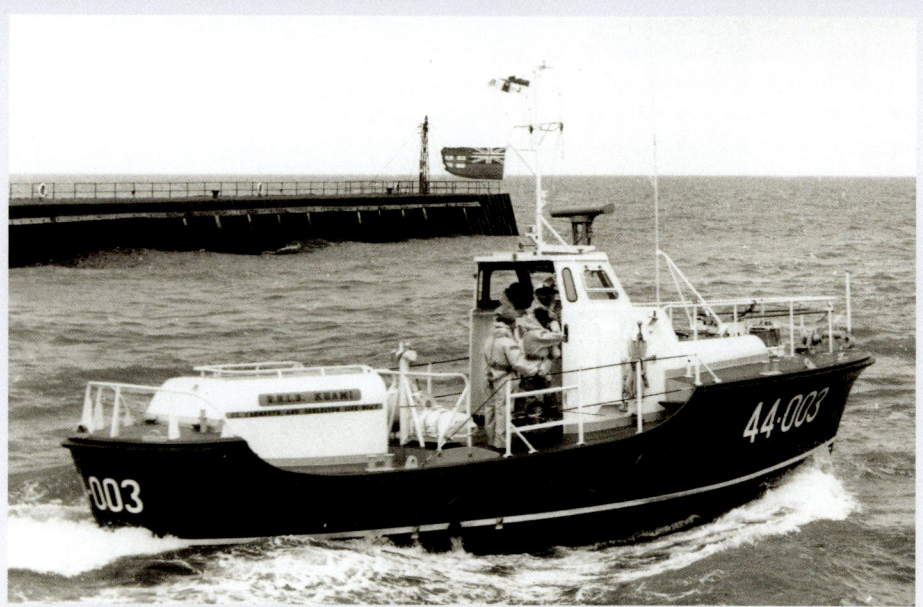

▲ 44-003 heading out of Gorleston harbour in the late 1960s, in her original pale grey livery.

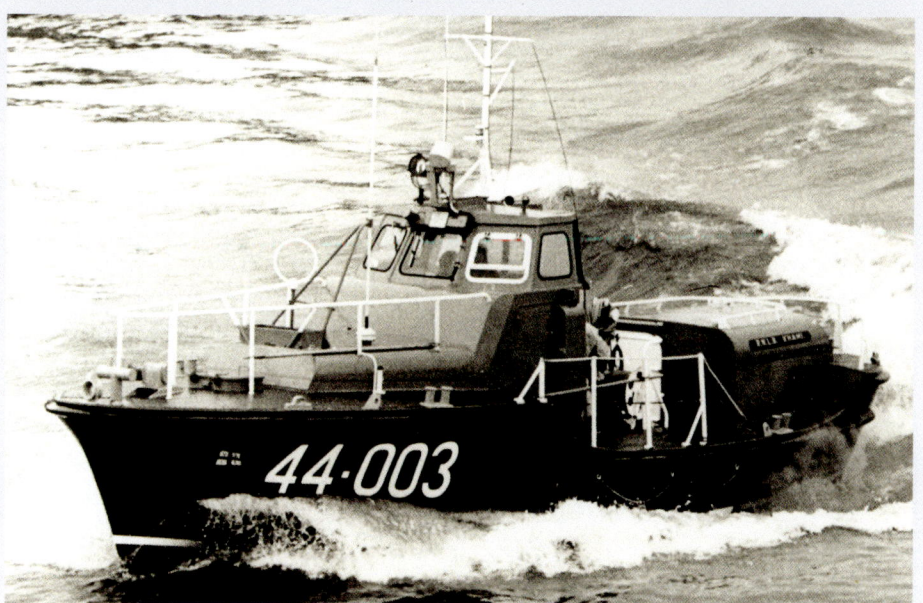

▲ 44-003 returning to Gorleston, wih her superstructure painted orange. (By courtesy of the RNLI)

Khami

▶ 44-003, while on station at Great Yarmouth and Gorleston, arriving at Carrow Bridge, Norwich, with kidney patients stranded by heavy snow, February 1979. (Eastern Daily Press)

▼ 44-003 at Harwich, moored at Navyard Wharf, while on relief duty, May 1995. (Nicholas Leach)

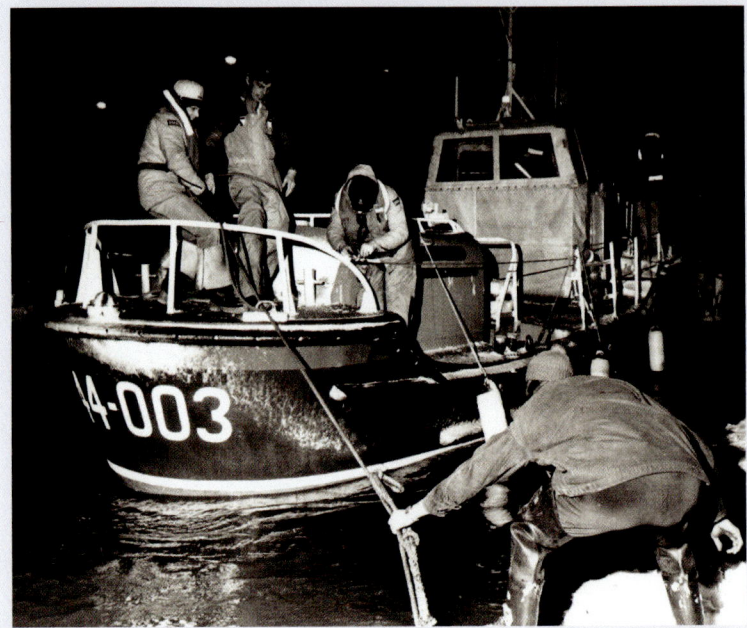

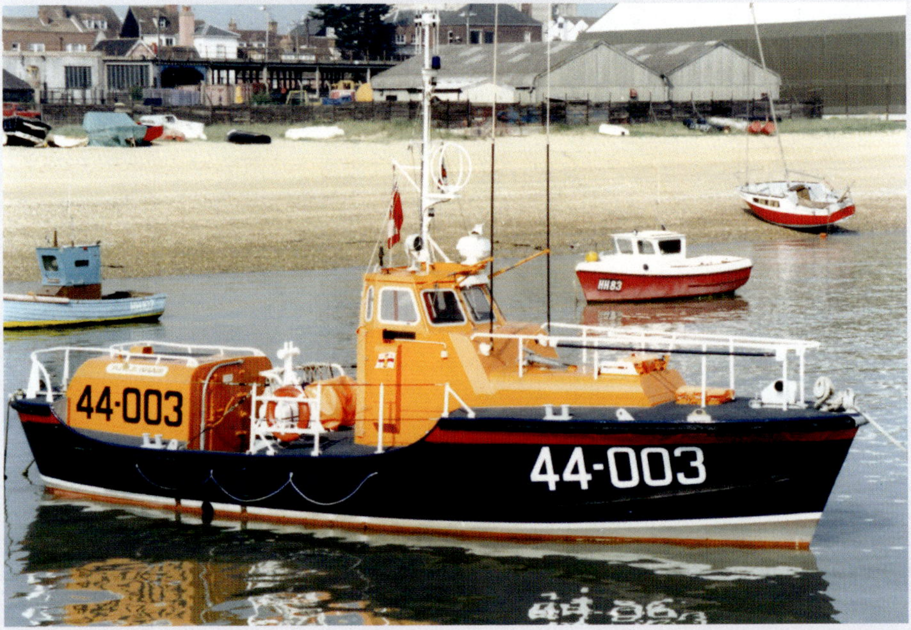

WAVENEY LIFEBOATS

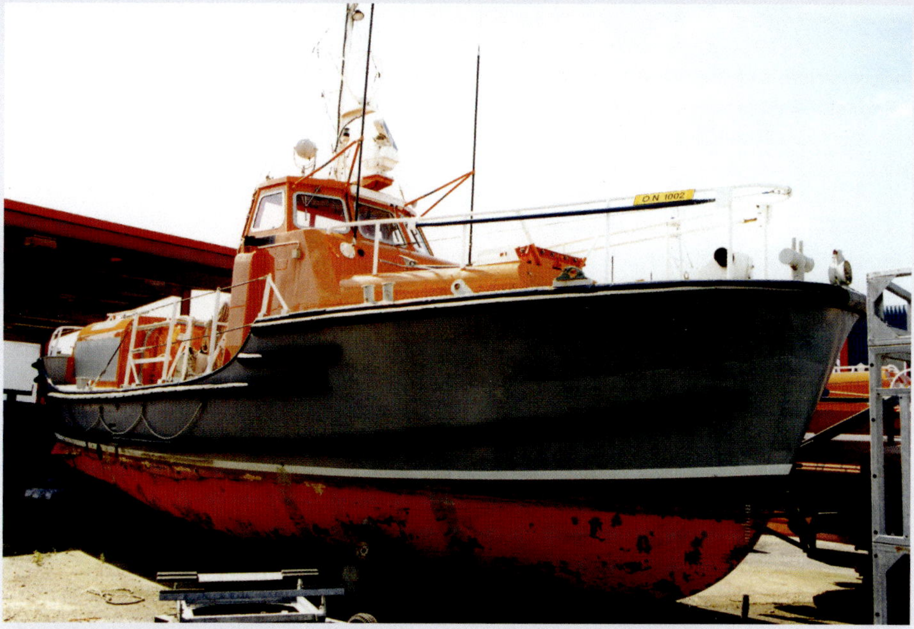

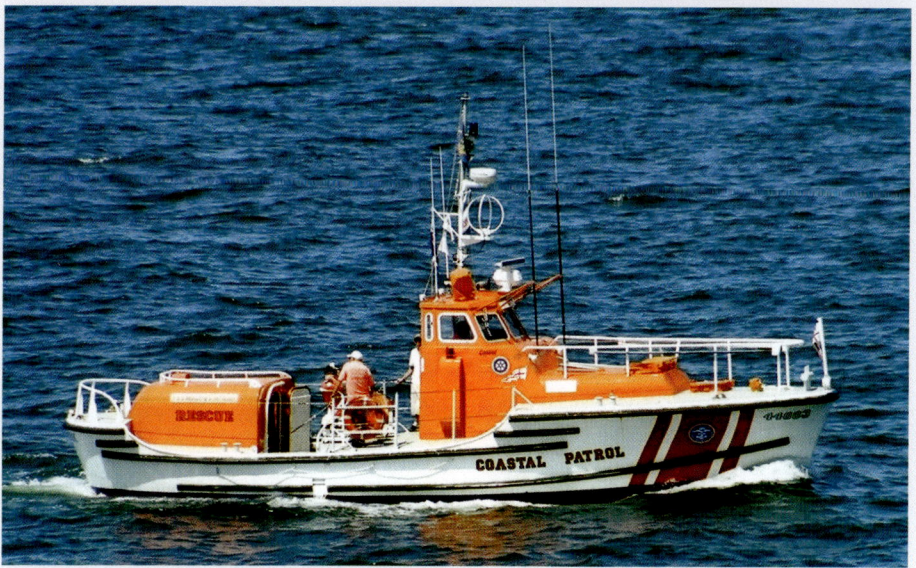

▲ 44-003 at the RNLI Depot, Poole, awaiting disposal, April 1999. (Nicholas Leach).

▲ 44-003 renamed P&O Nedlloyd Stratheden in service with the RVCP, Australia. (Mick Prendergast)

Faithful Forester

Key data

Built 1967, Brooke Marine, Lowestoft; yard no. B350
Donor Ancient Order of Foresters; the eighth boat donated by the Order in the 20th century
Named 26 Jul 1967 at Dover by HRH Princess Marina, Duchess of Kent
Stations Dover 26 Jul 1967 – 2 Oct 1979 (202/140), Relief 7 Oct 1979 – 11 Jun 1984 (49/18),
Holyhead 12 Jun 1984 – 14 Sep 1985 (25/26), Relief 14 Sep 1985 – 27 Jun 1997 (98/28)
Disposal Sold 21 May 1999 to Royal Volunteer Coastal Patrol, Australia

Service career

Faithful Forester served at Dover for twelve years, and then spent a further sixteen years
in the Relief Fleet, which included a stint at Holyhead that lasted more than a year. During
her time at Dover, she undertook many services, including a particularly challenging one on
1 December 1975. Under the command of Coxswain Arthur Liddon, she was launched to
help the 1,199-ton coaster Primrose, of Cyprus, which was in difficulty in force ten winds. The
severe weather was creating appalling conditions at the harbour entrance and, while clearing
the harbour, the lifeboat was laid on her beam ends but righted herself and carried on. She
then stood by the casualty, which was shipping heavy seas, while the crew on Primrose rigged
makeshift steering gear enabling the vessel to slowly make headway. When two miles off the
harbour, the casualty's master requested a pilot, but as the pilot vessel could not leave her
berth in the dreadful conditions, the lifeboat acted as a guide, taking station ahead of the
coaster and leading her to a berth. In recognition of the fine seamanship shown by Coxswain
Liddon during this rescue, he was awarded the Silver medal; the Bronze medal was awarded to
Second Coxswain Anthony Hawkins and the Thanks Inscribed on Vellum was accorded to the
remainder of the crew, Assistant Mechanic Richard Hawkins, John Smith and Gordon David.

While in the Relief Fleet, Faithful Forester served at many stations, including St Helier in the
Channel Islands, where she was involved in an outstanding service on 14 December 1982 to
the yacht Festina Lente III, of Norway. The yacht's engine and steering gear had failed when
the yacht was a mile south of St Helier Harbour entrance. In force six winds the lifeboat,
under the command of Coxswain Michael Berry, encountered moderate to rough seas as she
made her way out of the harbour, quickly finding the casualty, which had been deep within
an outcrop of rocks. Without hesitation, having quickly assessed the situation, Coxswain Berry
took the lifeboat into an area of heavily broken water to get to the casualty. As there was
no possibility of towing the yacht to safety, the Coxswain instructed her two crew to leap on
board the lifeboat as he placed the lifeboat's starboard side alongside to the yacht. He then

executed a skilful withdrawal, stern first as there was not enough room to turn the lifeboat. The rescue had taken only five minutes, but two lives had been saved. For this rescue, the Bronze medal was awarded to Coxswain Berry; Medal service certificates were presented to the remainder of the crew: Acting Second Coxswain David Aubert, Mechanic Dennis Aubert, Emergency Mechanic David Mills, William Hibbs and John Gray.

After service

Faithful Forester was placed on the sale list on 3 May 1997 and sold out of service on 21 May 1999 to the Royal Volunteer Coastal Patrol, Australia, for service in the Narooma Division as a Coast Guard vessel and lifeboat. Repainted in Coastal Patrol livery (white hull) at Souter Shipyard, Cowes, she was kept at the RNLI Depot, Poole, until being shipped to Australia. She arrived in Australia on 10 November 1999 and was renamed P&O Nedlloyd Strathmore. In April 2011, after serving Narooma for more than ten years, she was taken out of service, although she had not been used for more than a year due to mechanical problems. She was sold to Harbour Services Australia in Fremantle, and taken by road to Western Australia. After being refurbished, she was used in Fremantle Harbour as a crew transfer and utility vessel, renamed Harbour Conquest, with her aft cabin removed. In November 2017 she was sold for AUS$79,000 to another new owner, who undertook an extensive refit at Fremantle.

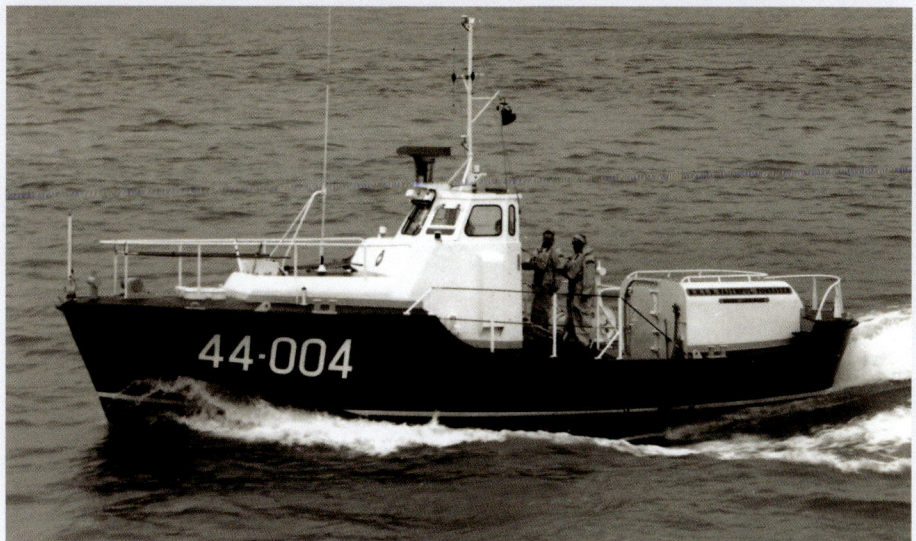

▲ 44-004 on exercise off Dover with her superstructure painted white, July 1967. (John G. Callis)

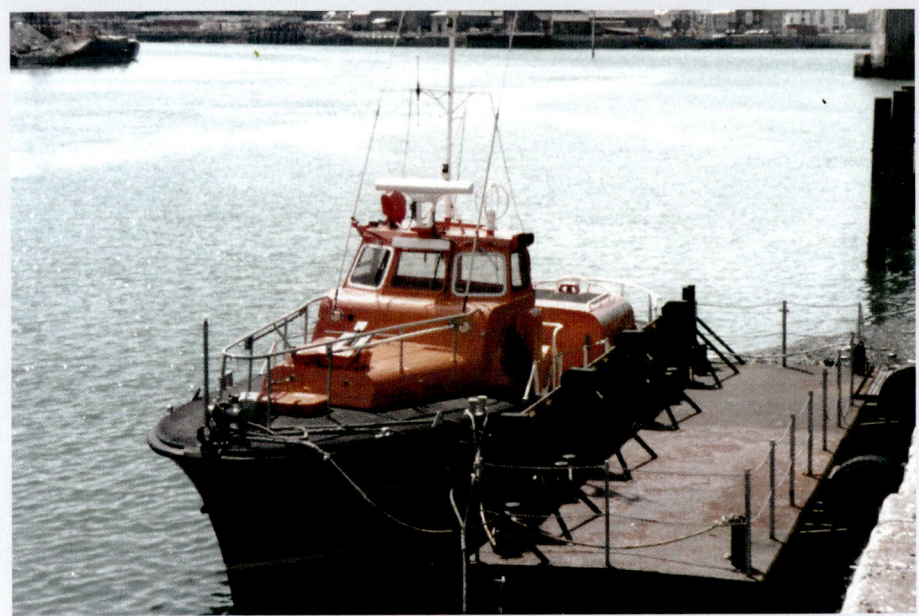

▲ 44-004 on temporary station duty at Holyhead, July 1984. (Tony Denton)

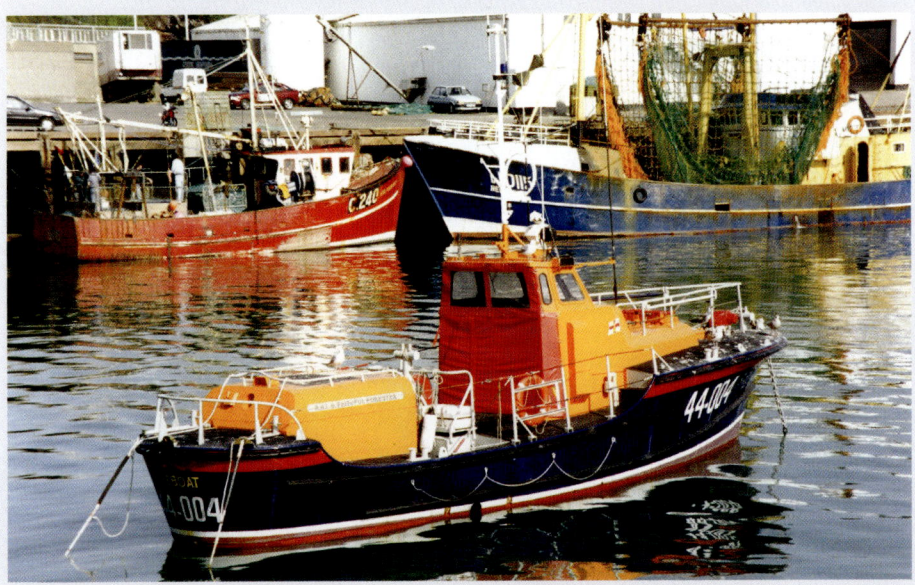

▲ 44-004 on relief duty at Dunmore East, April 1997. (Nicholas Leach)

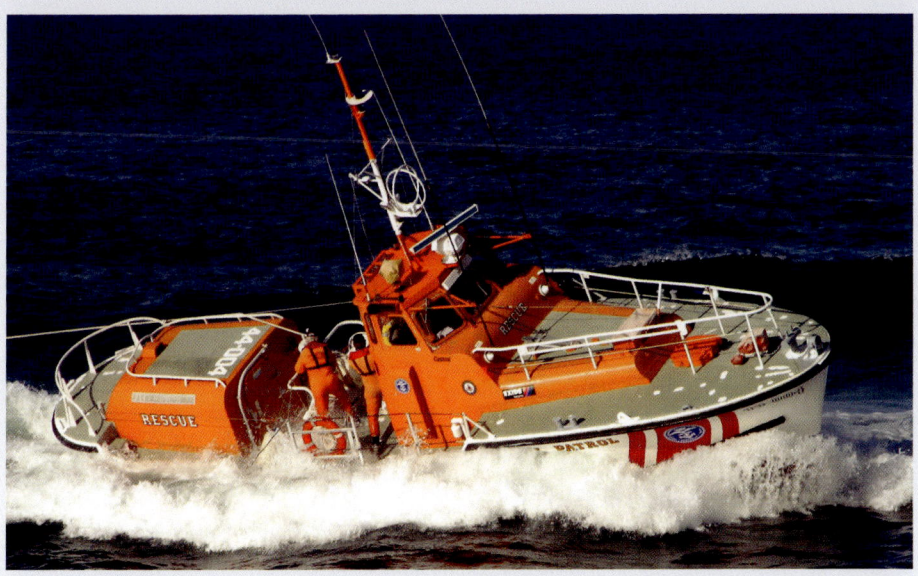

▲ 44-004 at Narooma in the colours of the Australian Coastal Patrol renamed P&O Nedlloyd Strathmore, 2003.

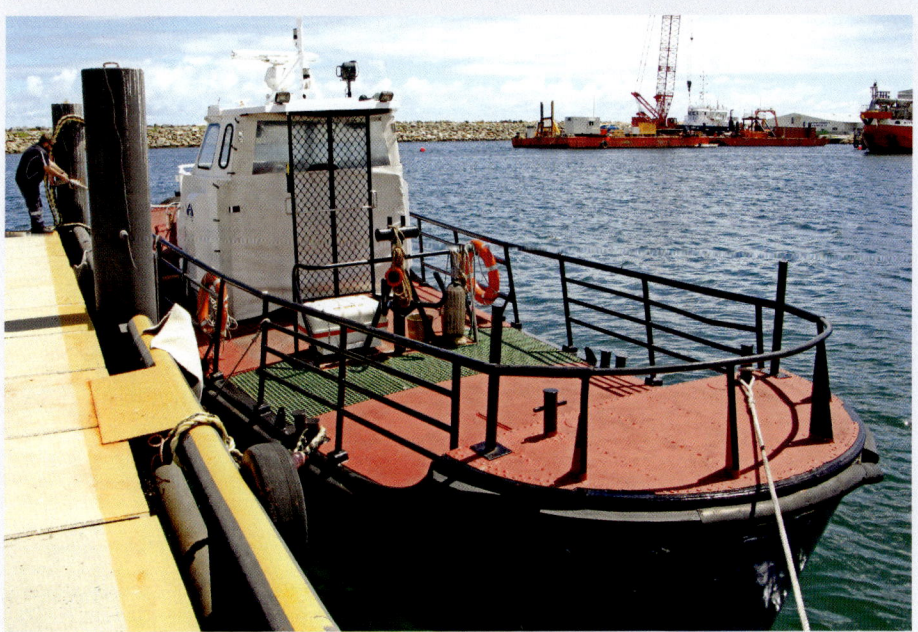

▲ 44-004 in Fremantle renamed Harbour Conquest with her aft cabin removed, October 2015.

Margaret Graham

Key data

Built 1967, Brooke Marine, Lowestoft; yard no. B351

Donor An anonymous gift to record the friendship of William H. Cavenaugh, Hazel M. Dugan, Theodore and Margaret N. Harley with the donor

Named 27 Sep 1967 at Trinity House Pier, Harwich, by Captain G.E. Barnard, deputy master of Trinity House.

Stations Harwich 27 Sep 1967 – Mar 1980 (173/77); Relief 1980 – Jun 1996 (49/14); Amble 9 Jun 1986 – Jul 1999 (164/6)

Disposal Sold 4 Aug 1999 to Scarborough Borough Council (Whitby Harbour Board)

Service career

Margaret Graham arrived at Harwich in September 1967 and served the station for almost thirteen years, before being transferred to the Relief Fleet. On 18 June 1972 she spent twelve hours chasing the 40ft ketch-rigged yacht Golden Miller. The yacht had fired a distress flare because she had engine trouble and was unable to slow down or turn into the wind when forty miles off Harwich. The lifeboat was called out and, while two ferries stood by, a dredger, coaster and tug also went to help, but none could get alongside the yacht because it was making seven knots and could not slow down in the strong winds. Margaret Graham crashed through the heavy seas but was unable to make much more than eleven knots in her pursuit of the yacht, so would be slow to arrive at the casualty. Great Yarmouth and Gorleston lifeboat Khami was also launched and she eventually reached the yacht and brought it into Lowestoft. Margaret Graham returned to Harwich after a round trip of 140 miles. Two of Golden Miller's crew were taken taken to hospital suffering severe seasickness. As a Relief boat, she served at a number of stations, including Dun Laoghaire, Donaghadee, Fleetwood and Troon. Her longest relief duty was at Dunmore East, from February 1984 to January 1985, during which time she was launched ten times on service. In June 1986 she was reallocated to Amble, in Northumberland, replacing a 37ft 6in Rother class lifeboat. She spent thirteen years at Amble, and, when replaced in July 1999, she was the last Waveney in RNLI operational service.

After service

Margaret Graham was replaced at Amble on 22 July 1999, placed on the sale list on 30 July 1999 and sold out of service on 4 August 1999 to Scarborough Borough Council. Renamed St Hilda of Whitby, she has been used as a pilot boat by Whitby Harbour Board, based at Whitby.

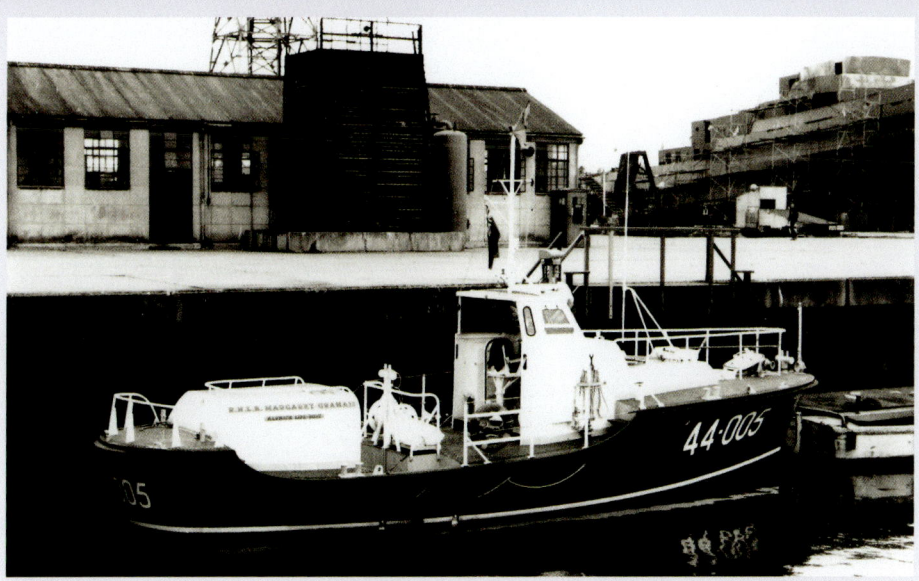

▲ 44-005 at Brooke Marine, Lowestoft, shortly after she had been completed, August 1967. (Jeff Morris)

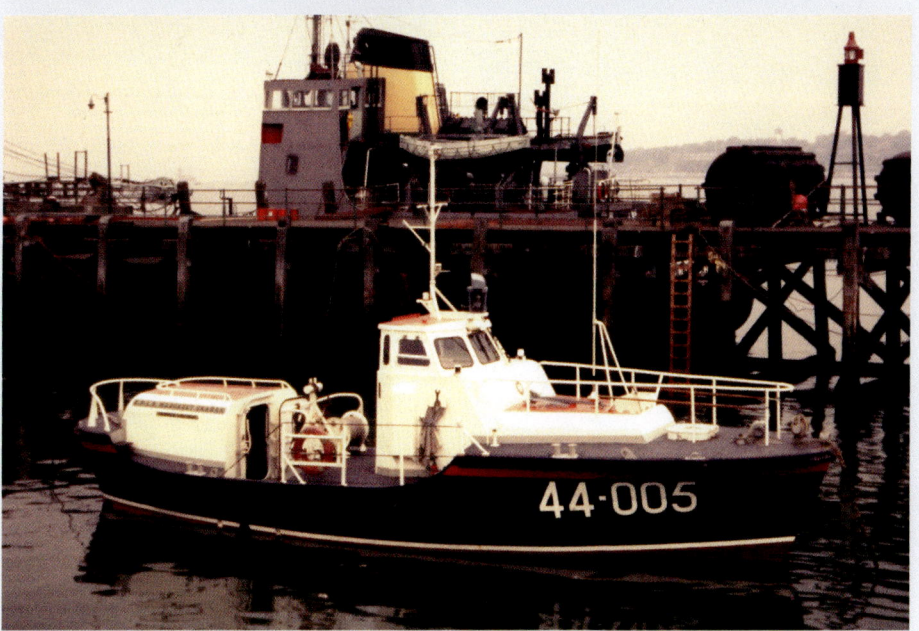

▲ 44-005 at Harwich, where she was usually kept at moorings in The Pound, near Halfpenny Pier. (RNLI)

Margaret Graham

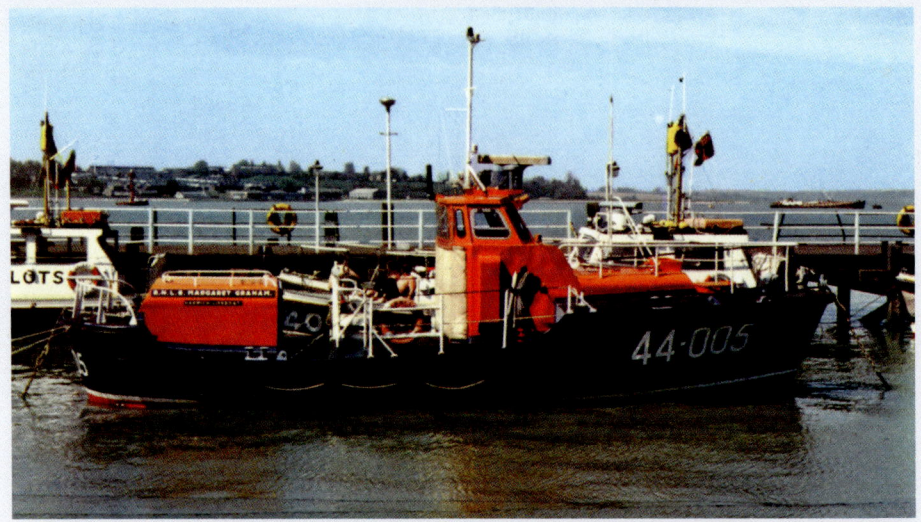

▲ 44-005 moored in the Pound at Harwich, after the superstructure colour was changed from white to orange.

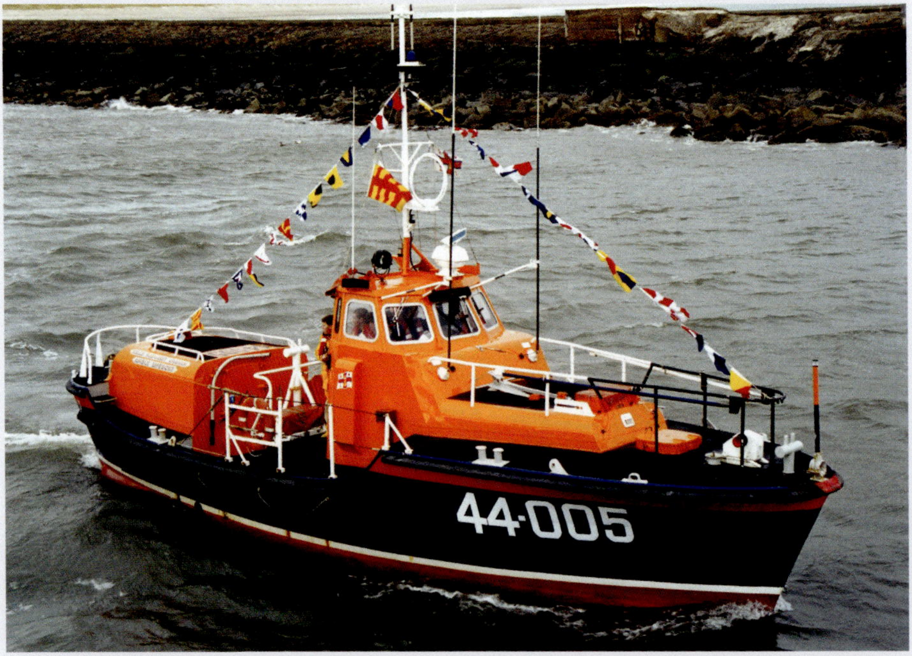

▲ 44-005 departing Amble harbour to attend a naming ceremony at Craster, March 1999. (Nicholas Leach)

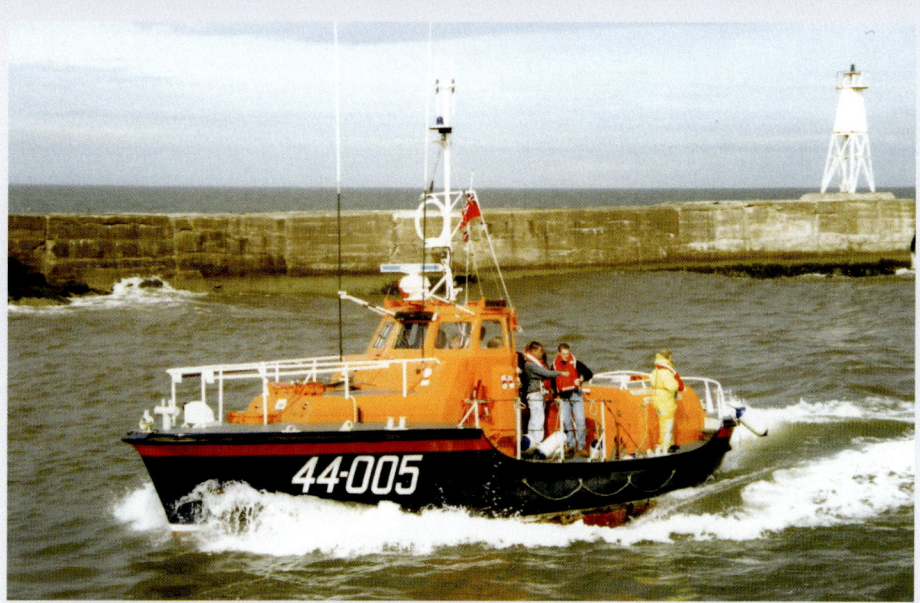

▲ 44-005 entering Amble harbour. (Steve Dutton)

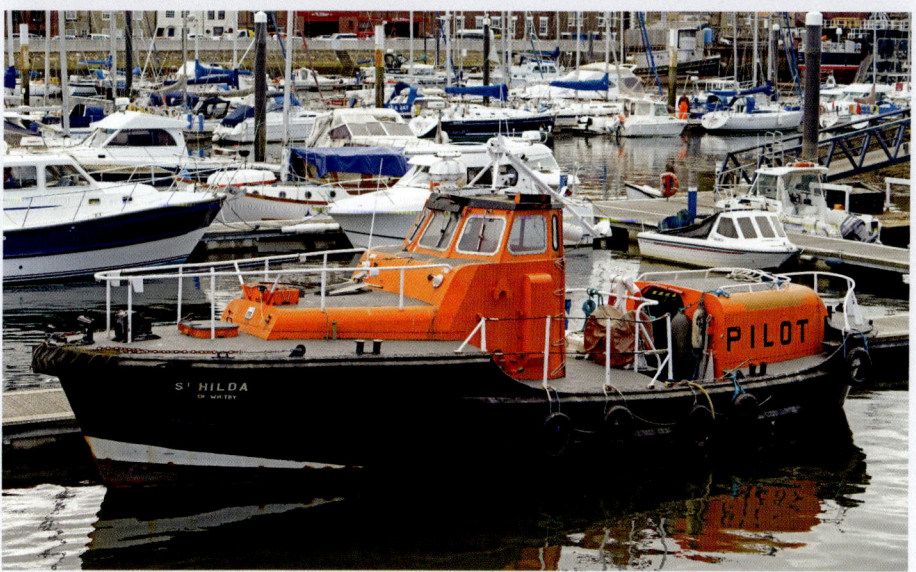

▲ 44-005 was sold out of service to Scarborough Borough Council and renamed St Hilda of Whitby. Pictured at Whitby in July 2020, she was used as a pilot boat, remaining largely unaltered. (Nicholas Leach)

Arthur and Blanche Harris

Key data

Built 1967, Brooke Marine, Lowestoft; yard no. B352

Donor Legacy of Mrs B.A.L. Harris, London

Named 2 May 1970 at Barry Dock by Lady Traherne, wife of the Lord Lieut of Glamorganshire

Stations Barry Dock 14 Mar 1968 – 7 Jun 1974 (109/44), Relief Jun 1974 – Aug 1979 (33/7), Donaghadee 23 Aug 1979 – Dec 1985 (8/43), Relief 1985 – 1993 (56/18), Courtmacsherry Harbour May 1993 – Sept 1995 (17/7), Relief 1995 – 1996 (2/0)

Disposal Sold 21 May 1999 to Royal Volunteer Coastal Patrol, Australia.

Service career

Arthur and Blanche Harris arrived at Barry Dock in March 1968 and spent just over six years at the South Wales station, before being replaced by an Arun. She then had a varied career, serving as a relief lifeboat as well as having longer stints at Donaghadee and Courtmacsherry Harbour. The most notable rescue performed by Arthur and Blanche Harris took place on 14 September 1987 when she was on relief duty at Fleetwood. She was launched under the command of Coxswain William Fairclough at 8.50pm to the fishing vessel Galilean, of Penzance, which was taking in water five miles west of Blackpool. In force six winds and rough seas, the lifeboat was laid over on her beam ends on two occasions, but, once she reached the casualty, a tow line was secured and for two hours the tow was maintained despite the heavy seas. However, shortly after midnight the fishing vessel became unstable with a large amount of water in her hull, so the two crew abandoned her, got into their liferaft and were taken onboard the lifeboat which stood by until the fishing vessel sank. The lifeboat then returned to Fleetwood to land the survivors. For this service, the Thanks Inscribed on Vellum was accorded to Coxswain Fairclough, and vellum service certificates went to the rest of the crew.

After service

Arthur and Blanche Harris was sold out of service on 21 May 1999 to the Royal Volunteer Coastal Patrol, Australia, for service as a coastguard vessel and lifeboat in the Ulladulla Division. Stored at the RNLI Depot, Poole, until being shipped to Australia, she was repainted in the Coastal Patrol colours (white hull) and renamed P&O Nedlloyd Strathallan (after the ship that transported her). In 2007 she was replaced by ON.1058 (an ex-RNLI Arun) at Ulladulla and reallocated to Broken Bay Division, Bayview, New South Wales. In 2009 she was sold to Harbour Services Australia, renamed Harbour Crusader, and joined ex-ON.1060 to augment their fleet in Fremantle. After ten years in Fremantle, she was scrapped in 2019.

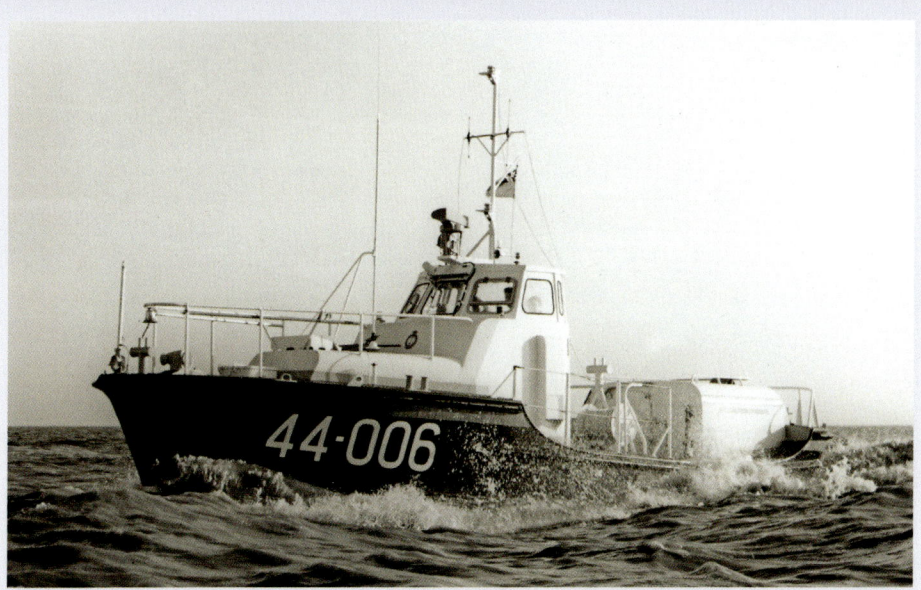

▲ 44-006 on trials off the Suffolk coast in 1967, prior to entering service. (Author's collection)

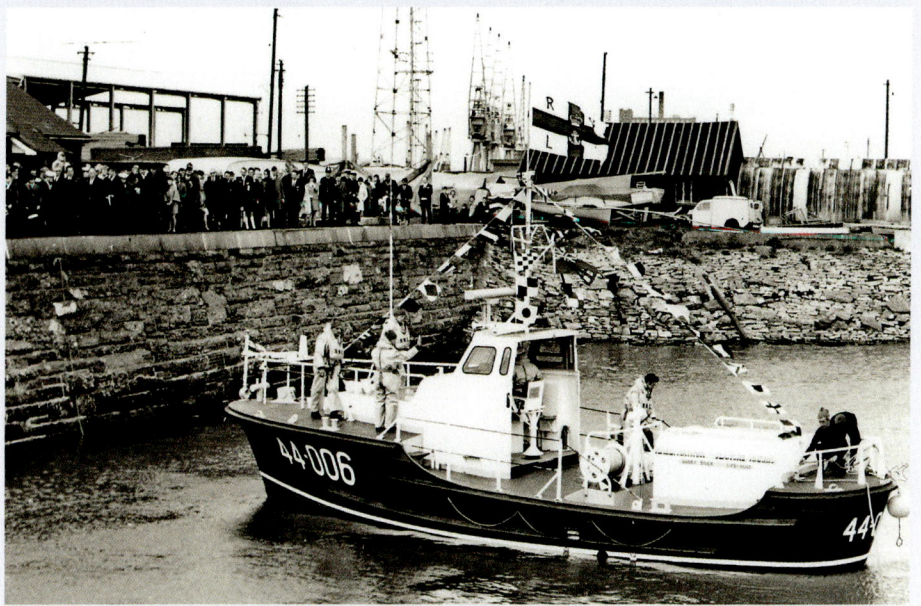

▲ 44-006 during her naming ceremony at Barry Dock on 2 May 1970. (Jeff Morris)

WAVENEY LIFEBOATS

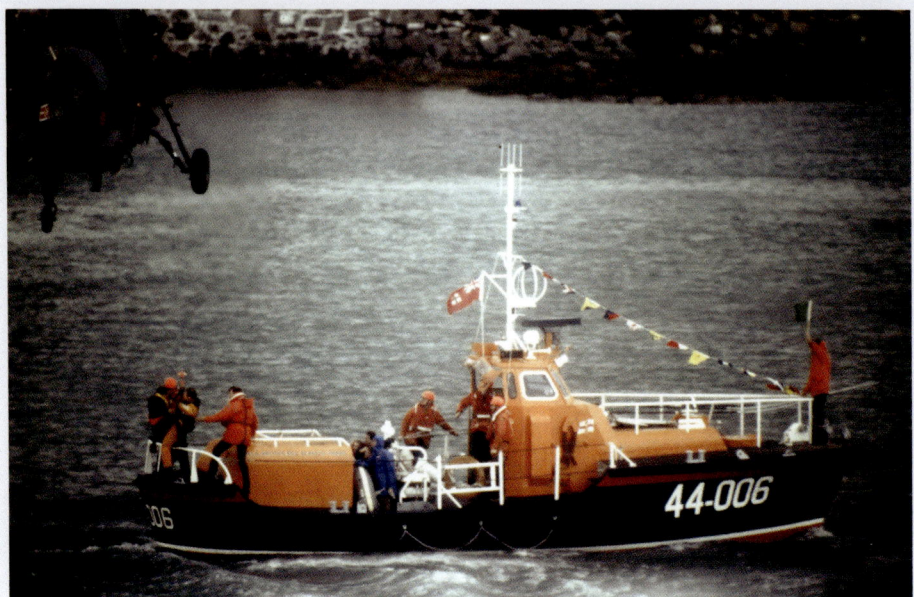

▲ 44-006 on exercise with an Army helicopter at Donaghadee, Co Down, August 1985. (Colin Watson)

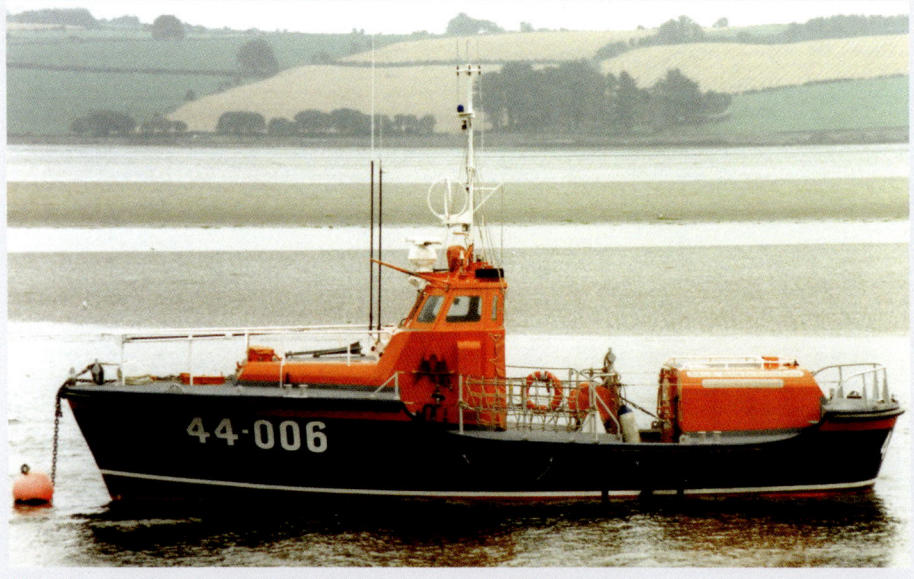

▲ 44-006 moored at Courtmacsherry Harbour, August 1995. (Nicholas Leach)

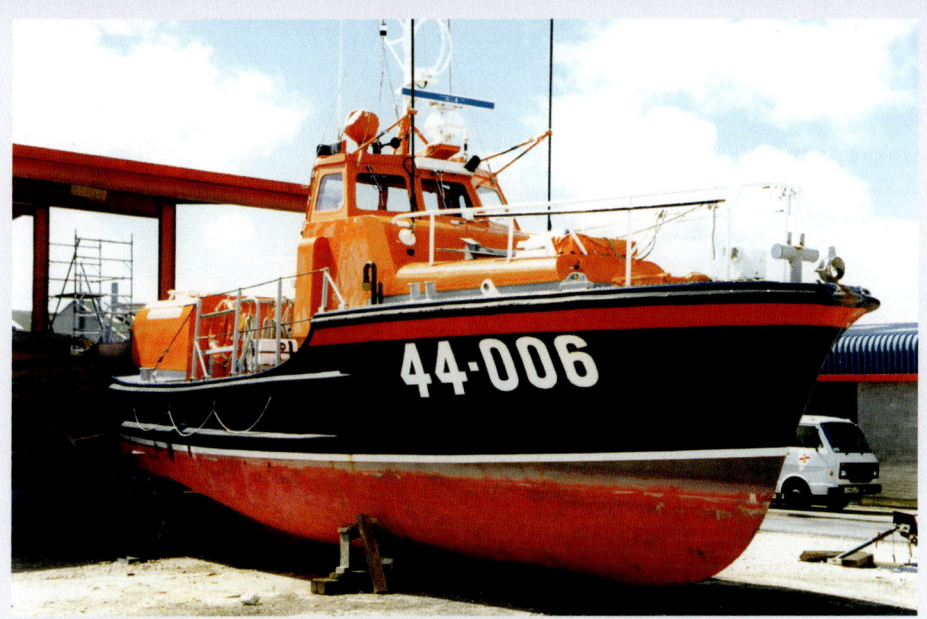

▲ 44-006 awaiting disposal at the RNLI Depot, Poole, July 1996. (Nicholas Leach).

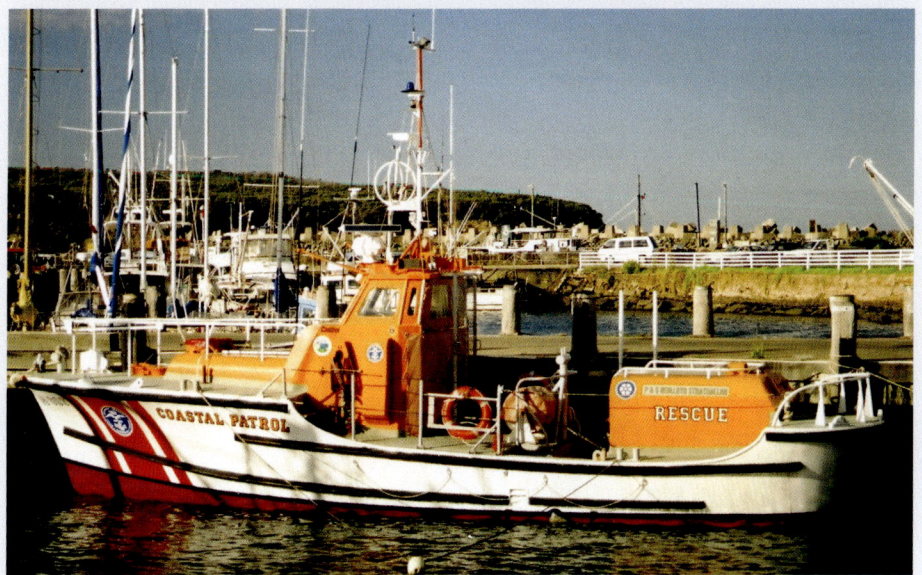

▲ 44-006 renamed P&O Nedlloyd Strathallan at Ulladulla, Australia.

Connel Elizabeth Cargill

Key data

Built 1967, Brooke Marine, Lowestoft; yard no. B353

Donor Legacy of the late W.A. Cargill, Carruth, Bridge of Weir, in memory of his mother

Named 5 Oct 1968 at Troon by Mrs Connel Leggatt

Stations Troon Aug 1968 – Aug 1985 (45/66), Arklow 7 Mar 1986 – June 1990 (29/19), Relief 1990 – 1997 (33/3)

Disposal Sold 14 May 1999 to Royal Volunteer Coastal Patrol, Australia

Service career

Connel Elizabeth Cargill spent seventeen years on station at Troon, where she was involved in a significant service on 12 September 1980 to the dredger Holland I (see page 50). She was involved in another fine service on 18 October 1984, going to the fishing vessel Golden Years, with a crew of three, which was in difficulty a mile off Irvine in exceptionally heavy seas and and force eleven south-westerly storm, with winds gusting up to 100mph. The lifeboat and her crew quickly reached the casualty and towed her clear of the shore and heavy surf. A second line was passed across by the lifeboat crew and the lifeboat towed the disabled vessel into Troon. For this excellent service, Acting Coxswain Thomas Devenny was accorded the Thanks Inscribed on Vellum by the RNLI, with vellum service certificates being presented to the rest of the crew. After Troon, Connel Elizabeth Cargill served at Arklow for just over three years, before entering the Relief Fleet in 1990. During her seven years as a relief lifeboat, she was on temporary station duty at Portree during 1991 when that station was being established. She was used for crew training by Portree volunteers during early 1991, and was taken on passage to Portree in February 1991. She served on relief at many stations, including Invergordon, Montrose, Dunbar, Blyth and Eyemouth.

After service

Connel Elizabeth Cargill was sold out of service on 21 May 1999 to the Royal Volunteer Coastal Patrol, Australia, for use as a coastguard vessel and lifeboat in the Sydney Division. Repainted in the Coastal Patrol colours (white hull), she was shipped from Tilbury to Australia and renamed P&O Nedlloyd Rawalpindi (after the ship that transported her), being based at The Spit in Middle Harbour, Sydney. She was transferred to Marine Rescue NSW when that organisation came into being on 1 January 2010 as the only maritime rescue service in New South Wales. She was retired in December 2011 following a spell as a spare lifeboat at Middle Harbour Unit, Sydney Division, having been replaced by a new rescue boat. In early 2012 she was bought by a Brisbane-based owner and was on the Brisbane river used as a workboat.

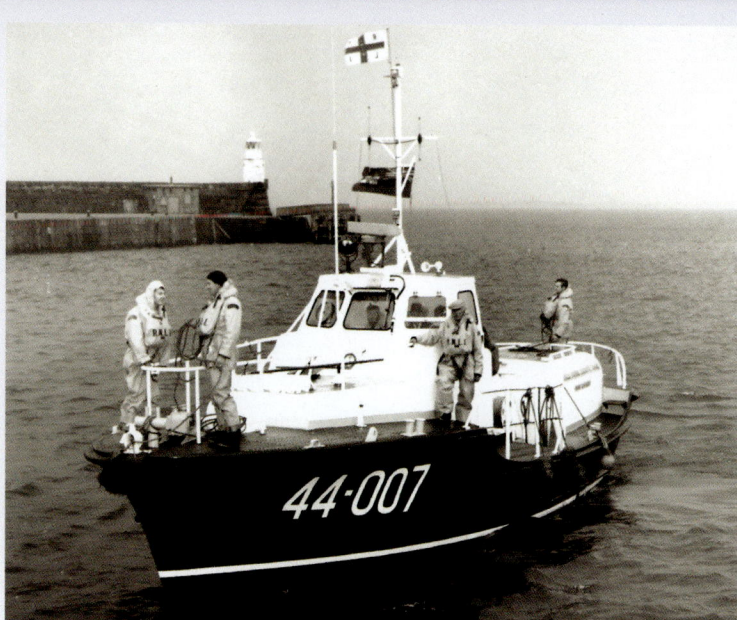

◀ 44-007, with white superstructure, approaches her berth after arriving at Troon. (Supplied by Ian Johnson)

▼ 44-007 approaching Troon harbour after her superstructure had been repainted in the RNLI's orange livery. (Ian Johnson)

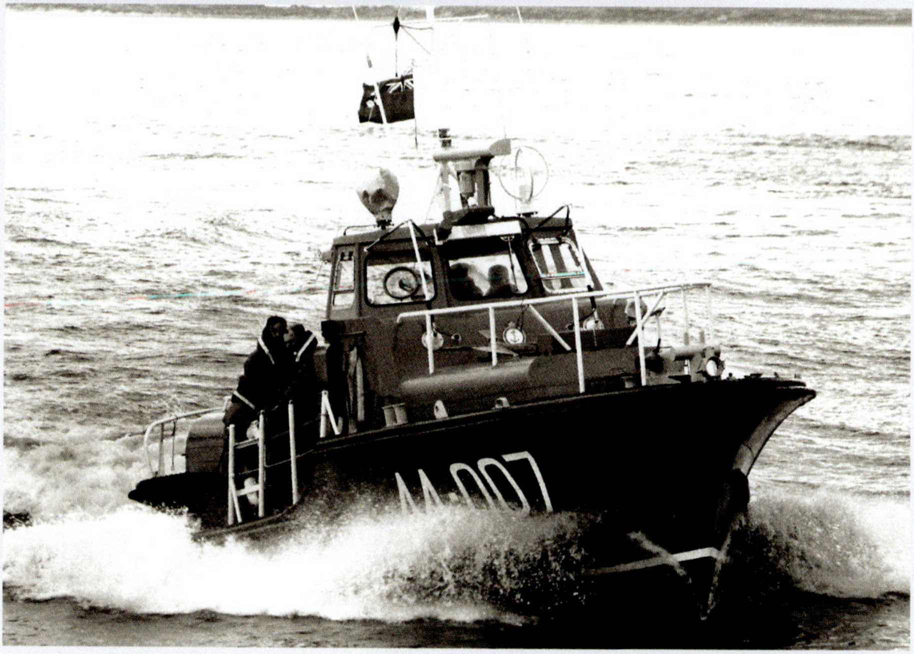

Connel Elizabeth Cargill

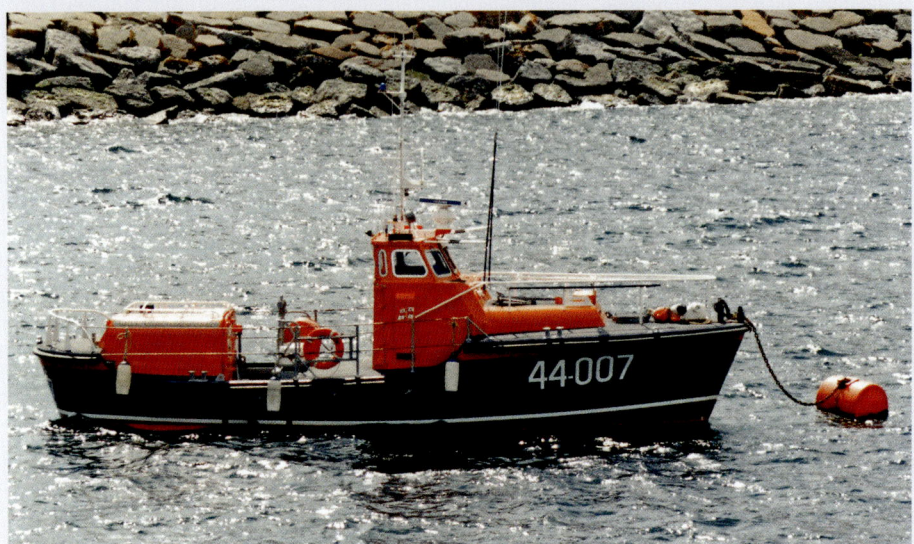

▲ 44-007 on relief at Dunbar, July 1994; she spent just over two months at the station in 1994. (Nicholas Leach)

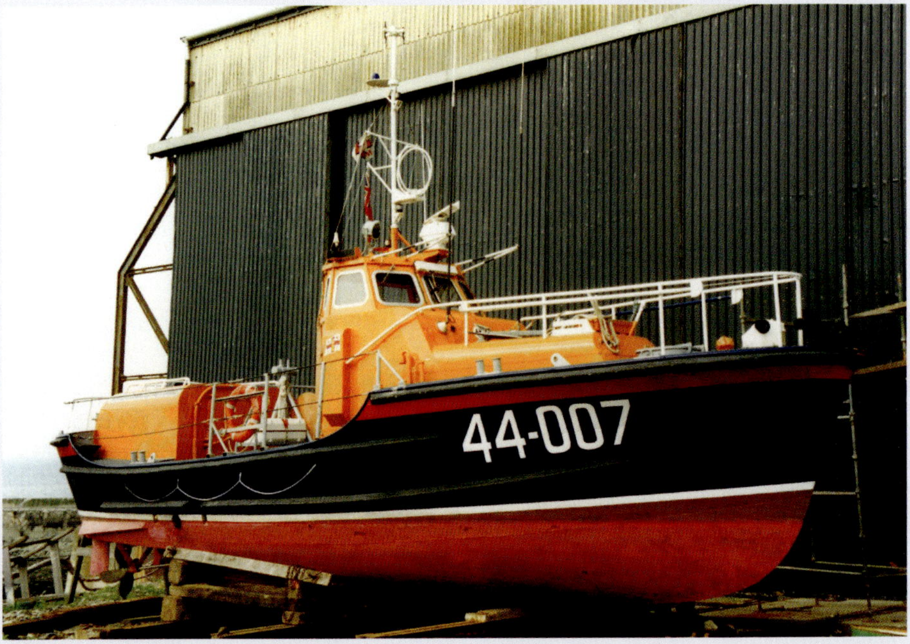

▲ 44-007 at Buckie Shipyard, Buckie, August 1997. (Nicholas Leach)

ON.1006 • 44-007

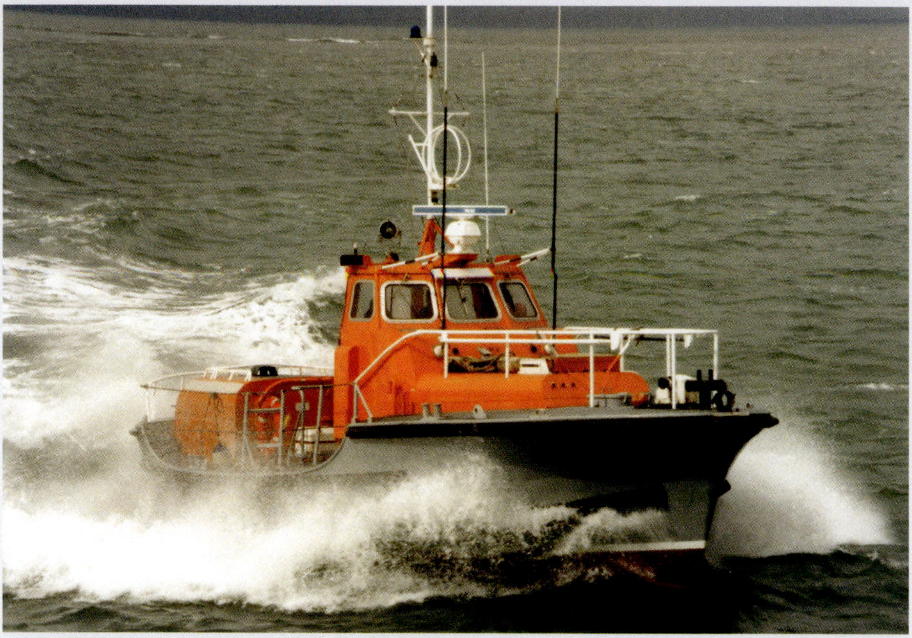

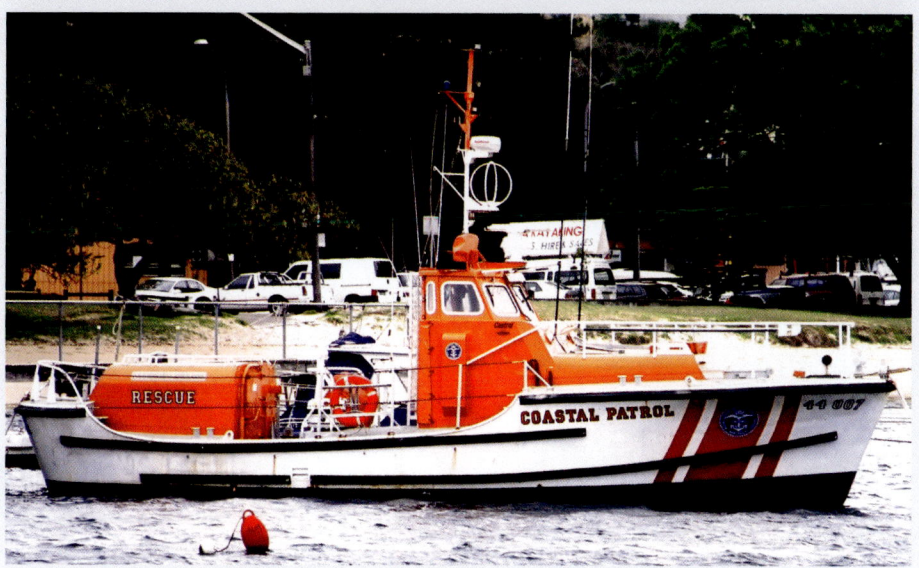

▲ 44-007, having been sold out of service, on passage in the Western Solent. (Peter Edey)

▲ 44-007 renamed P&O Nedlloyd Rawalpindi and moored at Sydney in RVCP livery.

Eric Seal (Civil Service No.36)

Key data

Built 1974, Groves & Guttridge, Cowes, yard no. G&G 658

Donor Civil Service Lifeboat Fund

Named 3 August 1974 at Eyemouth by Lady Seal, in memory of Sir Eric Seal KBE CB, a former Vice-President of the RNLI and Chairman of the Civil Service Lifeboat Fund

Cost £81,864.31

Stations Eyemouth 7 Feb 1974 – Mar 1996 (153/45)

Disposal Sold 27.7.1999 to Sea Rescue Institute of Namibia; the last Waveney sold by RNLI

Service career

Eric Seal (Civil Service No.36) spent her operational career at Eyemouth in the Scottish Borders, where she was stationed for more than twenty-two years, undertaking more than 150 rescues, including a particularly fine service in October 1992. The narrow entrance to Eyemouth Harbour could be difficult to negotiate in severe weather, and on 14 and 15 October 1992 it was closed to all shipping. However, despite this, Eric Seal (Civil Service No.8) put out to help the Tyne pilot launch Norman Forster, which had broken down with three people on board. Despite the difficult conditions at the harbour entrance, Coxswain John Johnston showed great skill, and used his knowledge of the narrow entrance, to get the lifeboat out and into deep water. Twice she struck the bottom as a heavy swell had built up at the harbour entrance. Big seas broke over her while she was en route to the casualty, which she reached at 11.38am. She was taken close enough to the launch for a tow line to be rigged, but returning to Eyemouth was impossible, so Coxswain Johnston headed north. The lifeboat eventually arrived at Port Seton, on the Firth of Forth, at 3.05pm where the casualty was berthed. The lifeboat was unable to return to Eyemouth as conditions at the harbour entrance were so bad, so she made for Burnmouth, to the south. For this service, the Thanks Inscribed on Vellum was accorded to Coxswain Johnston in recognition of his skill, courage and outstanding leadership. Vellum service certificates were presented to the remainder of the crew: Second Coxswain/Mechanic James Tarvit, Acting Assistant Mechanic David Collin and crew members John Buchan, John Purves and Robert Aitchison.

After service

Eric Seal (Civil Service No.36) was placed on the sale list on 18 May 1996, sold out of service in April 2000 and shipped to Walvis Bay, Namibia, for use as a lifeboat, being renamed Spirit of Standard Bank. In 2005 she was moved from Walvis Bay to Lüderitz.

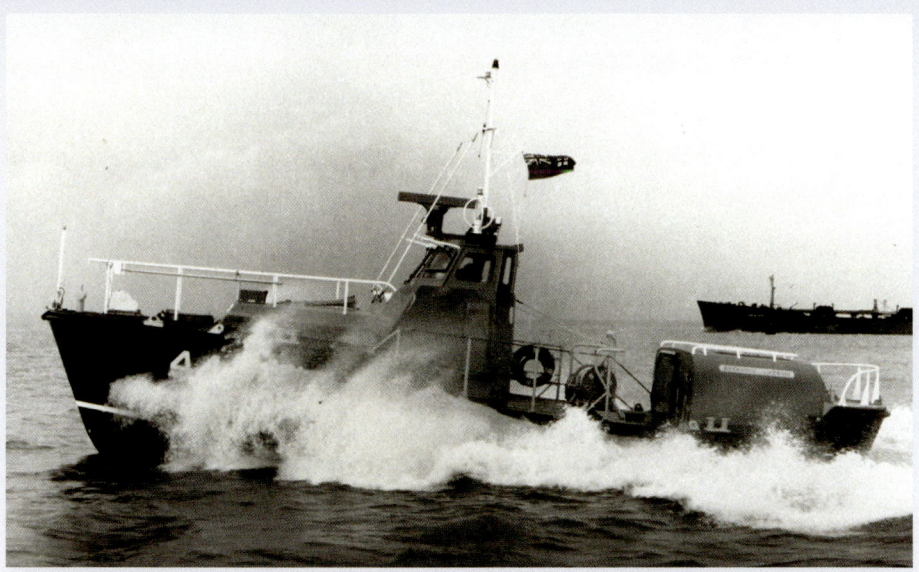

▲ 44-008 on acceptance trials prior to going on station at Eyemouth. (By courtesy of the RNLI)

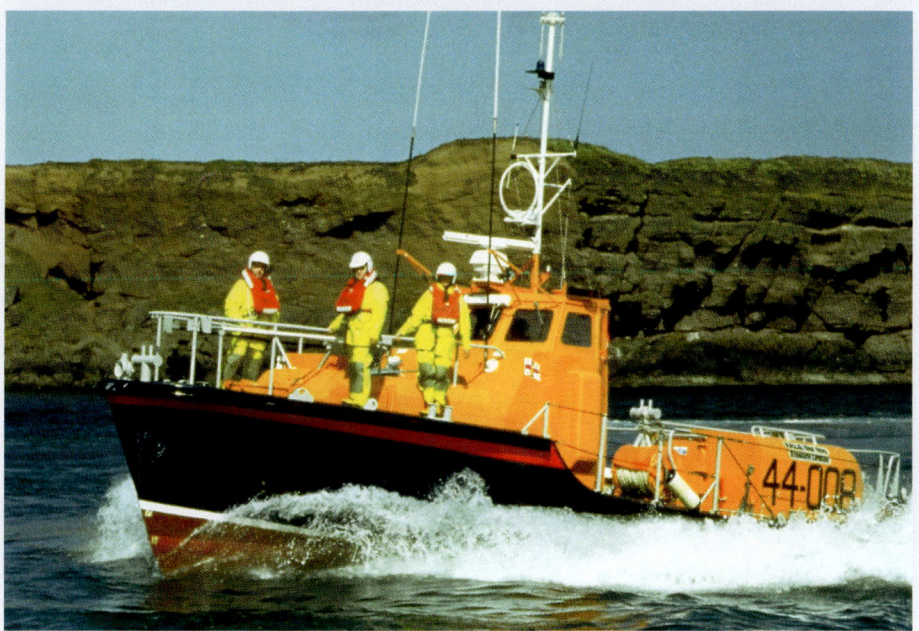

▲ 44-008 on station at Eyemouth. (By courtesy of the RNLI)

WAVENEY LIFEBOATS

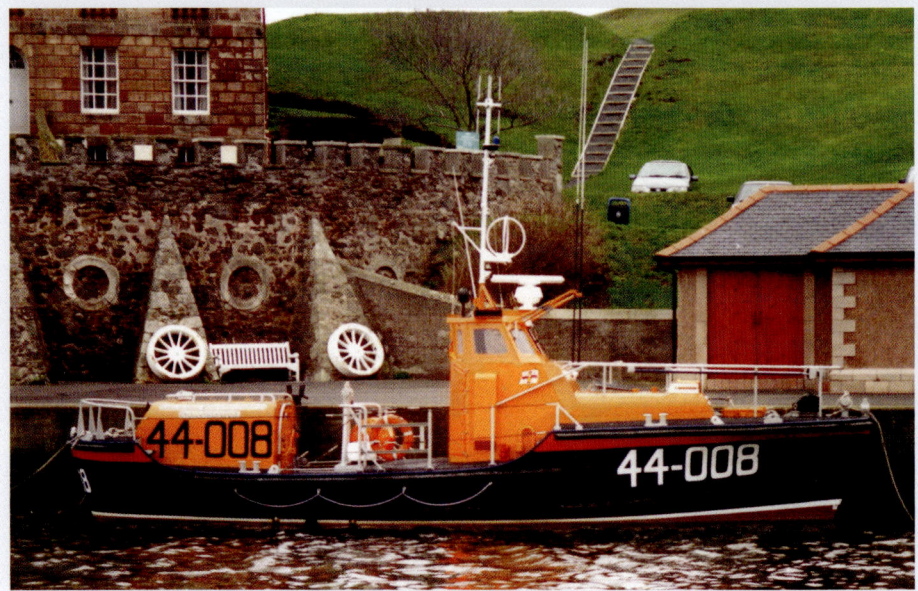

▲ 44-008 at her regular moorings at Eyemouth, 1995. (Richard Priest)

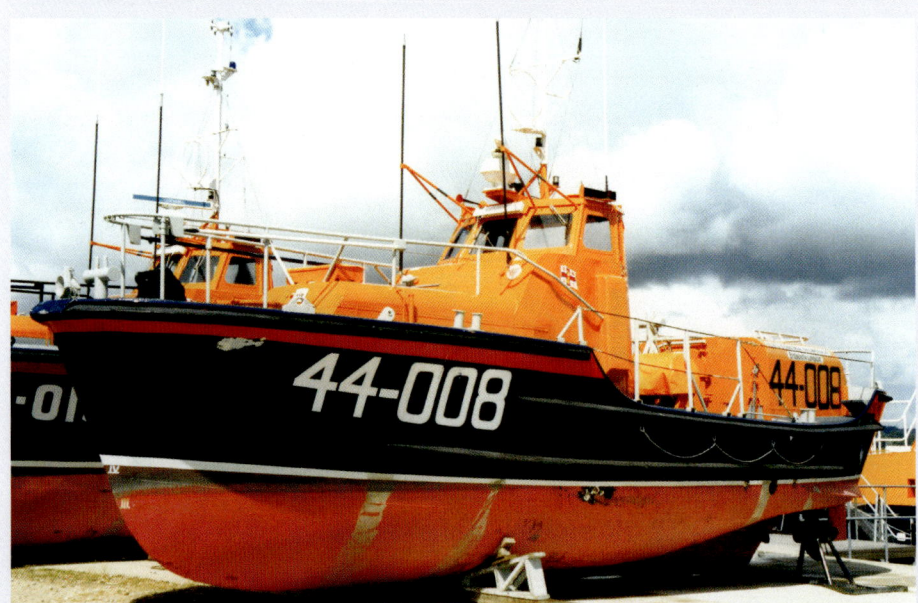

▲ 44-008 at the RNLI Depot, Poole, after being replaced at Eyemouth, July 1996. (Nicholas Leach)

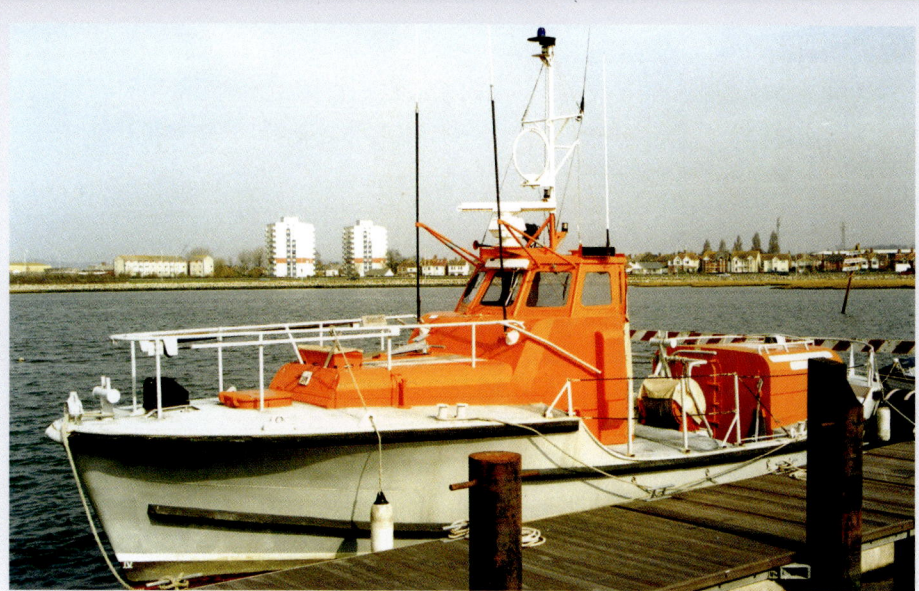

▲ 44-008 at the RNLI Depot, Poole, awaiting shipment to Namibia, March 2000. She was the last of the Waveneys to be sold out of service by the RNLI. (Nicholas Leach)

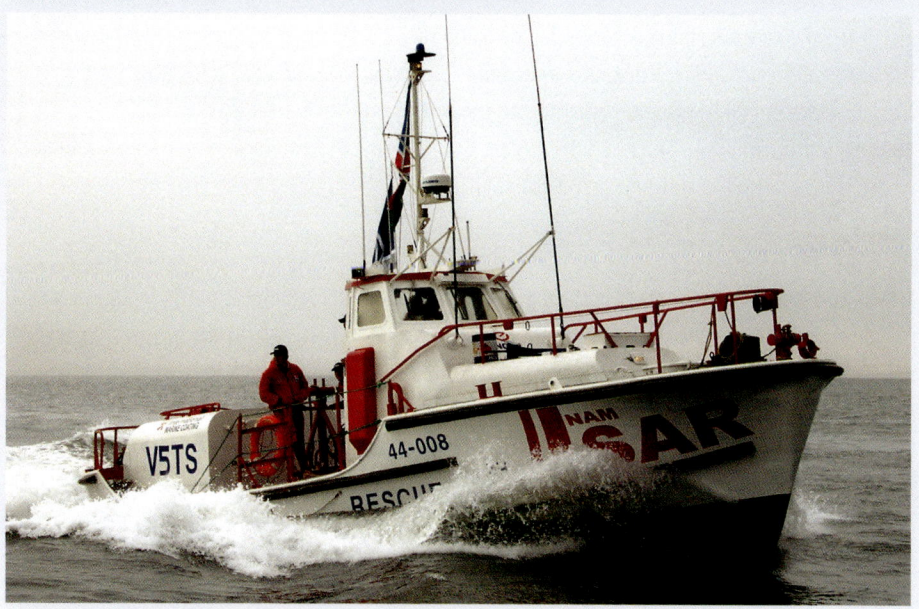

▲ 44-008 off Namibia, renamed Spirit of Standard Bank, September 2003. (Hilmar Snorrason/Iceship)

WAVENEY LIFEBOATS

Helen Turnbull

Key data

Built 1974, Groves & Guttridge, Cowes, yard no. G&G 659

Donor Legacy of James Bissell Turnbull, Ilfracombe; together with donations from Medway Lions Club and the Medway Lifeboat Appeal

Named 18 May 1974 at Sheerness Docks by Mrs R.D. Leigh-Pemberton

Cost £73,271.53

Stations Sheerness 4 Apr 1974 – Mar 1996 (649/297), Achill Island 28 Aug 1996 – Jan 1998 (9/0), Relief Jan 1998 – Nov 1998 (24/7)

Disposal Sold 20.11.1998 to Maurice Singer, Isle of Man

Service career

Helen Turnbull spent almost twenty-two years on station at Sheerness, where she was the station's first new lifeboat. During this time she was involved in many outstanding rescues for which her Coxswain was formally recognised by the RNLI. One of these took place on 30 December 1978, when she was launched in a severe gale (force nine), with rough breaking seas and frequent heavy snow flurries to the cabin cruiser Ma Jolie II, which had lost her propeller and was dragging her anchor. The lifeboat was taken through yacht moorings to get alongside the casualty, and succeeded in rescuing the cruiser's two occupants. For this service, the Bronze Second Service clasp was awarded to Coxswain/Mechanic Charles Bowry and medal service certificates were presented to the rest of the crew. After leaving Sheerness in 1996, Helen Turnbull was sent to Achill Island, County Mayo, to establish a new lifeboat station where she became the station's first lifeboat.

After service

Helen Turnbull was sold out of service in November 1998 to Elan Investments, Douglas, IOM. Renamed Badger, she was converted into a pleasure boat at Ramsey, on the Isle of Man, and subsequently kept at moorings in Port St Mary outer harbour. She was substantially altered for leisure use; the wheelhouse was enlarged and enclosed, and the whole superstructure was painted white. In September 1999, she was moved to Coburg Marina, Liverpool, for the winter but returned to the Isle of Man in spring 2000. She broke her moorings and was damaged in September 2000, being taken to Dickie's Boat Yard, Bangor, for repairs, which took more than two years. She then moved between Preston Marina, Lake Windermere and Douglas. She was sold in about 2014 and moved to the Forth & Clyde Canal ar Bowling, West Dunbartonshire, where she was kept at Bowling Basin, renamed Sturm.

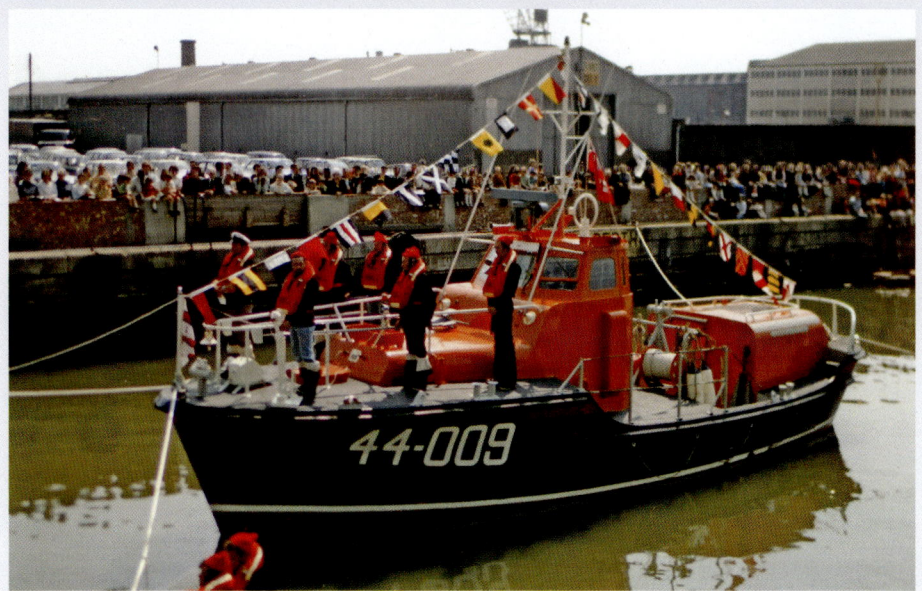

▲ 44-009 at Sheerness Docks for her naming ceremony of on 18 May 1974. She was christened by Mrs R.D. Leigh-Pemberton, wife of the vice Lord-Lieutenant of Kent. (Jeff Morris)

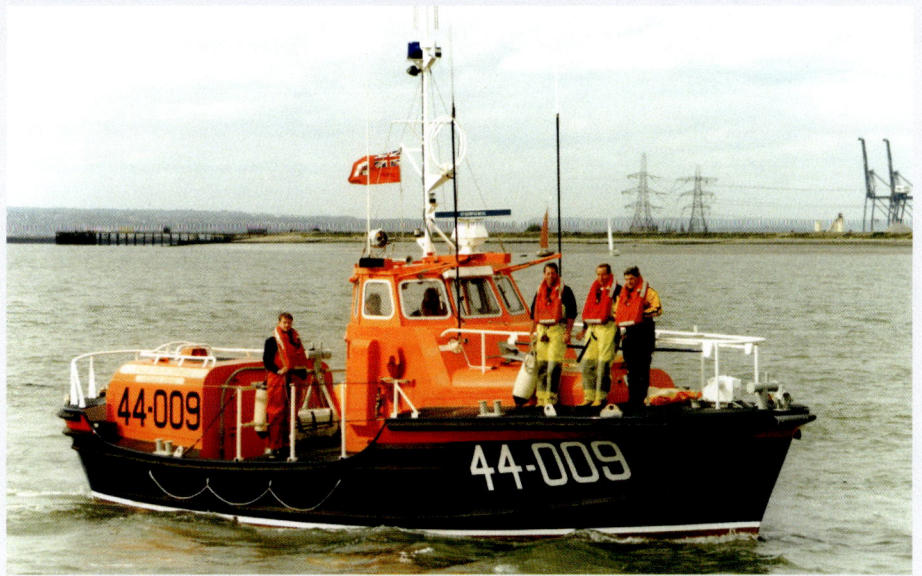

▲ 44-009 on exercise off Sheerness, September 1993. (Nicholas Leach)

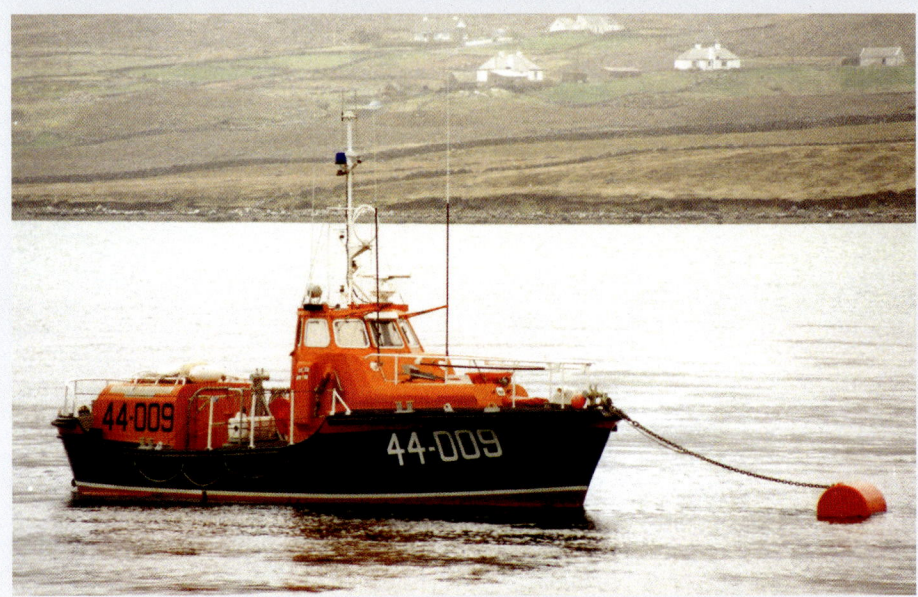

▲ 44-009 on station at Achill Island, moored in Achill Sound close to Kildavnet Pier, April 1997. (Nicholas Leach)

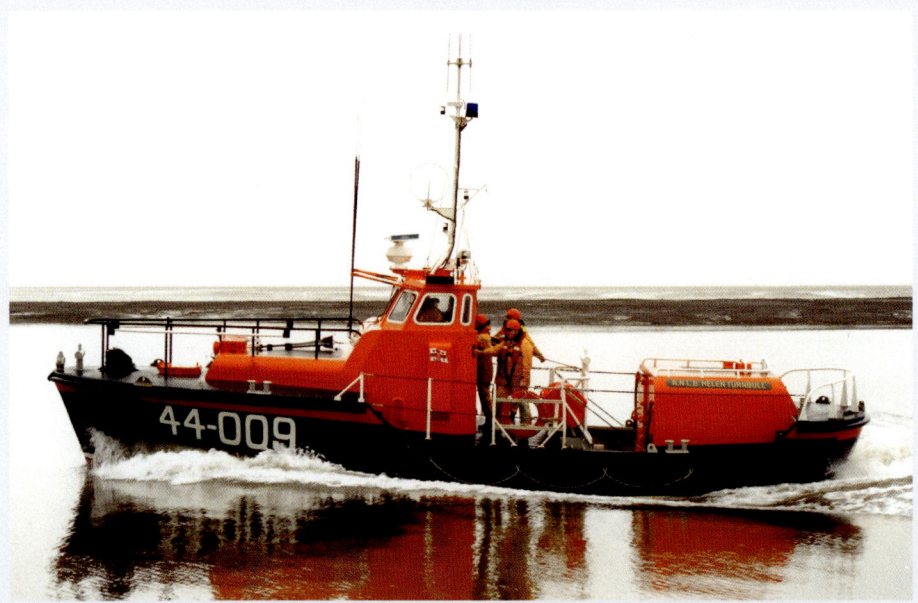

▲ 44-009 puts out on exercise while on relief duty at Fleetwood, February 1998. (Nicholas Leach)

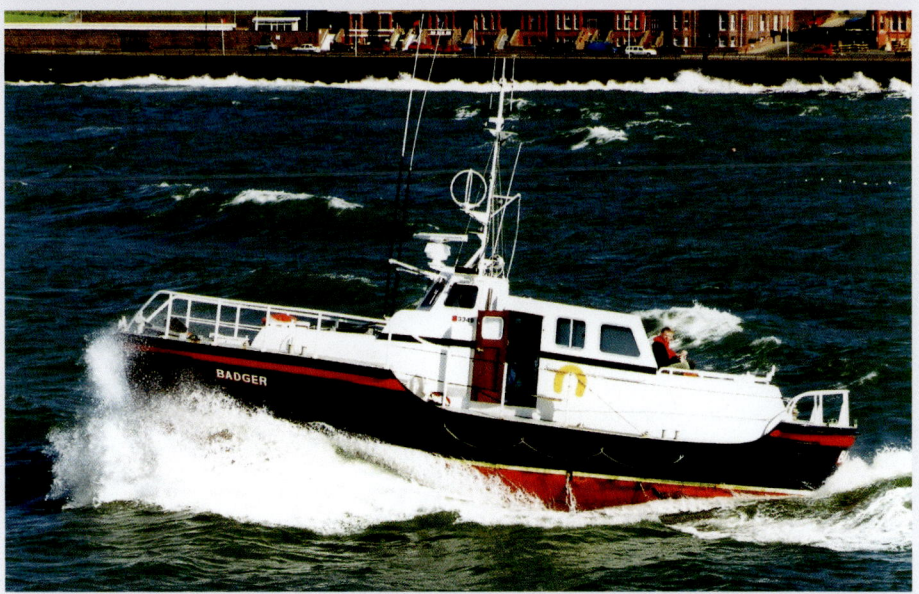

▲ 44-009 renamed Badger, in private ownership, departing Peel, Isle of Man, 2000. (Phil Weeks)

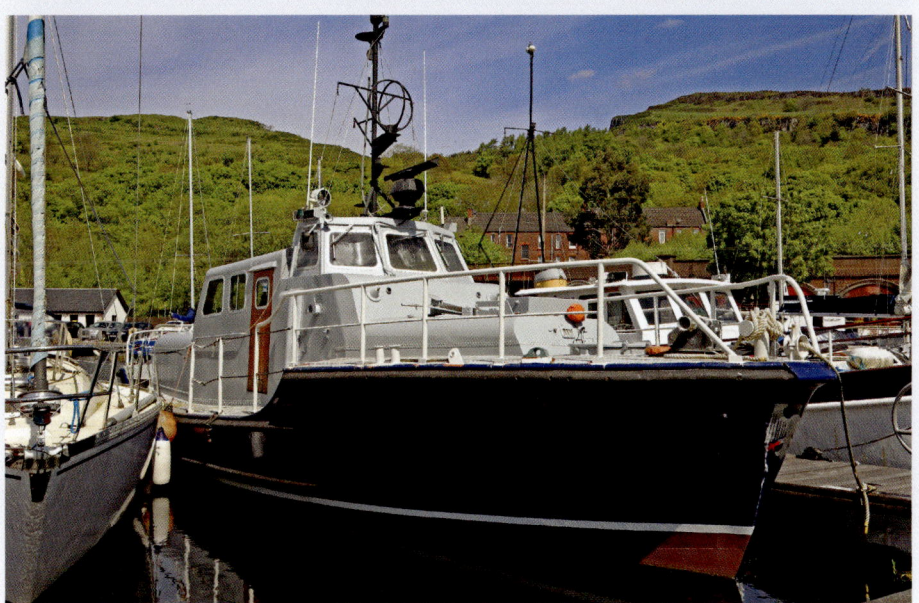

▲ 44-009 renamed Sturm at Bowling Basin, Bowling, West Dunbartonshire, May 2018. (Nicholas Leach)

Thomas Forehead and Mary Rowse II

Key data

Built 1974, Groves & Guttridge, Cowes, yard no. G&G 660
Donor Legacy of the late Thomas Field, Liverpool
Named 17 June 1975 at Millbay Docks, Plymouth, by the Duchess of Kent
Cost £68,736.94
Stations Plymouth 26 May 1974 –Sep 1987 (181/91); Fowey 26 Jan 1988 – Oct 1996 (169/35); Relief Oct 1996-1997 (4/0)
Disposal Sold 15.11.1999 to New Zealand Taranaki Volunteer Coastguard

Service career

Thomas Forehead and Mary Rowse II served at Plymouth for just over thirteen years, being replaced by a 52ft Arun and then reallocated to Fowey, where she served for more than eight years. Her most notable rescue was undertaken on 15 February 1978, when she was launched to the trawler Elly Gerda, of Teignmouth, which was in difficulty ten miles south west of Rame Head. The weather gradually worsened as the Waveney headed to the scene, and by the time the lifeboat reached the casualty the wind was severe gale force nine. The trawler had anchored east of Looe harbour to wait for the weather to improve, and the lifeboat stood by for several hours, with Acting Coxswain Patrick Marshall and Motor Mechanic Cyril Alcock taking turns at the helm. At 7.45pm the fishing vessel ran aground on rocks under a sheer cliff face. The sea was breaking over the nearby reef and the casualty, making the lifeboat's approach very hazardous. Acting Coxswain Marshall took the lifeboat alongside the fishing vessel twice, battling violent seas accompanied by heavy snow, and two men were taken off, leaving just the skipper on board. At one point, the lifeboat smashed down on the casualty, denting her bows but retained her watertight integrity. After a further two hours off the harbour entrance, the casualty entered escorted by the lifeboat. For this rescue, Bronze medals were awarded to Acting Coxswain Marshall and Mechanic Cyril Alcock.

After service

Thomas Forehead and Mary Rowse II was placed on the sale list on 3 December 1997 and sold out of service in 1999 to the Royal New Zealand Coastguard Federation. Renamed Westgate Rescue, she was used as a coastguard vessel and lifeboat operating from New Plymouth, Taranaki. In 2012 she was sold by the Coastguard to an owner in Picton, New Zealand, and was renamed Harrier. In 2015 she changed hands again, and in April 2019 was reported as being unaltered and being used in in Fiordland, New Zealand.

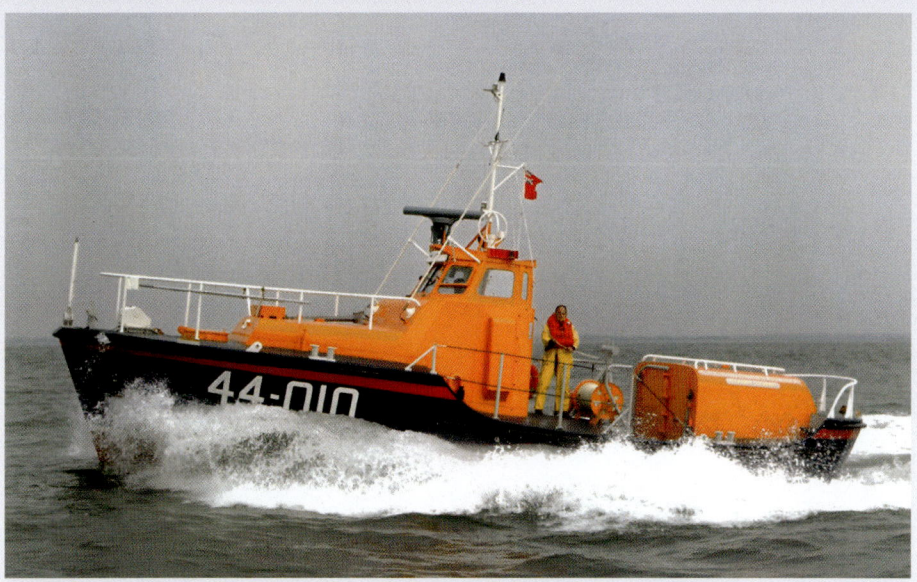

▲ 44-010 on trials prior to entering service. (By courtesy of the RNLI)

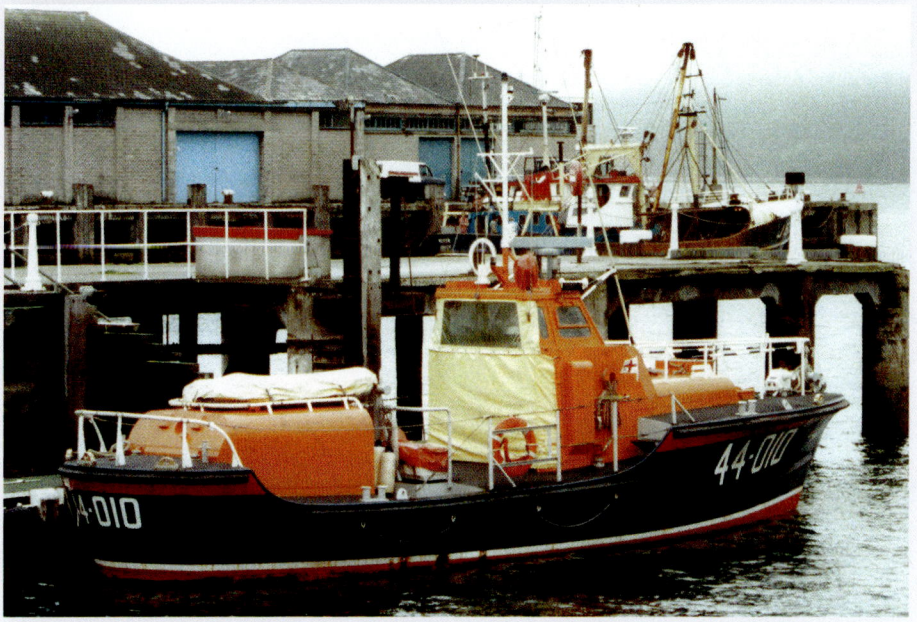

▲ 44-010 on station at Plymouth, moored in Millbay Docks. (Graham Brailey)

Thomas Forehead and Mary Rowse II

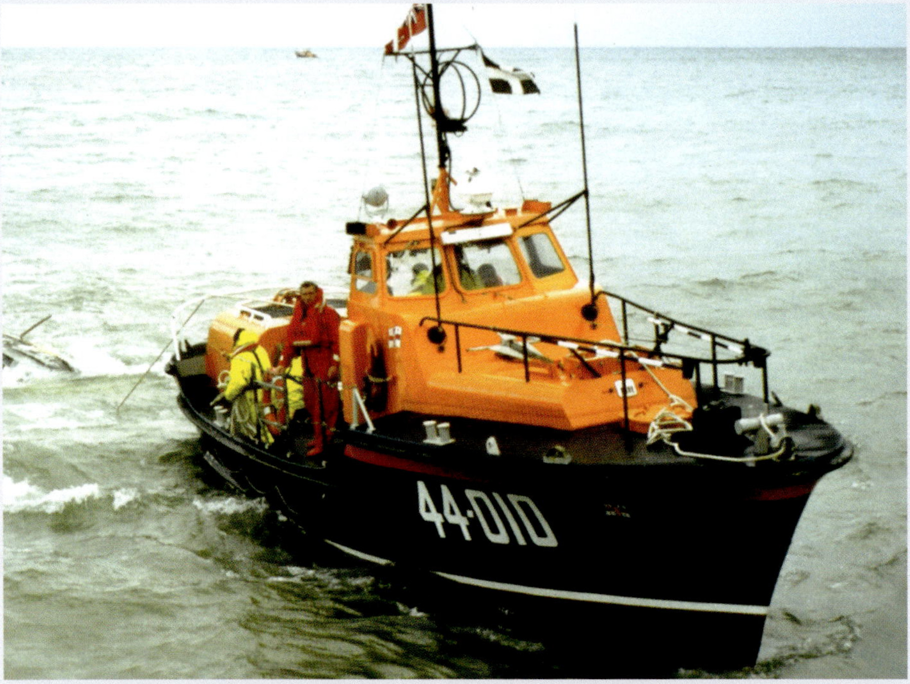

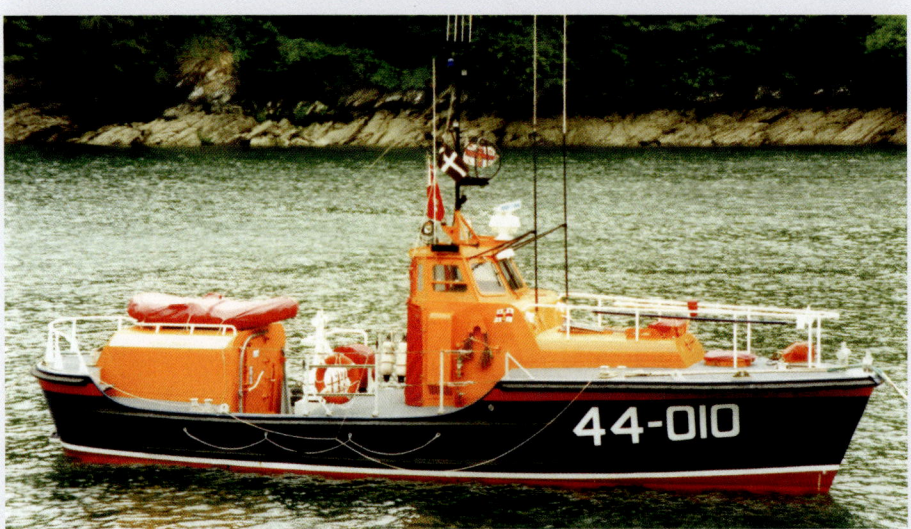

▲ 44-010 on service while she was stationed at Fowey. (By courtesy of the RNLI)

▲ 44-010 moored at Fowey, where she served for more than eight years, July 1996. (Nicholas Leach)

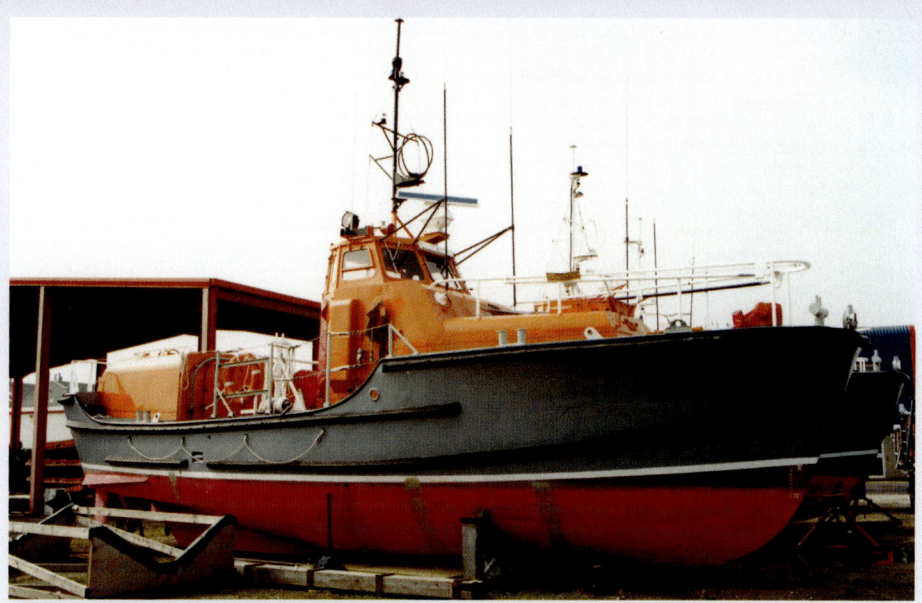

▲ 44-010 at the RNLI Depot, Poole, awaiting sale, September 1998. (Nicholas Leach)

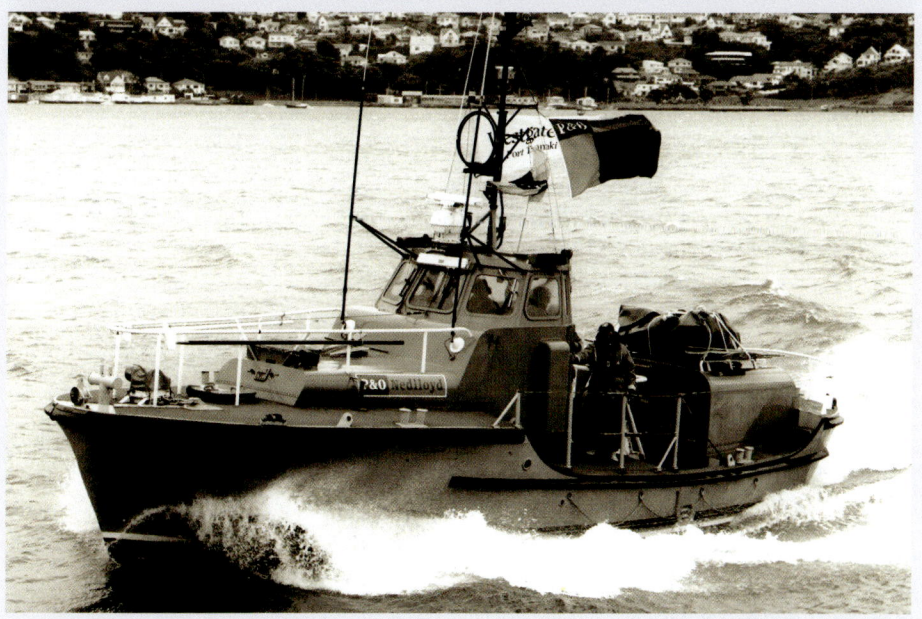

▲ 44-010, renamed Westgate Rescue, shortly after arriving in Wellington, New Zealand, 1999. (V.H. Young)

Augustine Courtauld

Key data

Built 1974, Groves & Guttridge, Cowes, yard no. G&G 661
Donor Gift of Mr W.P. Courtauld and the Mayor of Poole's Appeal
Named 7 May 1975 at Poole by Lady Rayner
Cost £68.736.32
Stations Poole Nov 1974 – Oct 1983 (106/32), Relief Oct 1983 – 1985 (8/5),
    Troon 25 Aug 1985 – Oct 1987 (53/38), Relief 29 Oct 1987 – 5 Jun 1990 (9/0),
    Arklow 5 June 1990 – Feb 1997 (78/26), stored at Poole 6 Apr 1997 – 10 May 1999 (1/1)
Disposal Sold 21 May 1999 to Royal Volunteer Coastal Patrol, Australia

Service career

Augustine Courtauld performed more than 100 services while she was stationed at Poole, many of which were routine. Some rescues, however, were more demanding, such as that undertaken on 8 January 1982. In blizzard conditions, with the wind blowing force ten and extremely rough seas, she was launched to the motor cruiser Trois Lions, which was in difficulty twelve miles south of Poole. During the passage to the casualty, Augustine Courtauld encountered heavy breaking seas in the Swash Channel. The casualty was found five miles south of Anvil Point. To make for Weymouth or Poole was considered too dangerous, so the lifeboat escorted the cruiser to Yarmouth, Isle of Wight, and, assisted by Yarmouth lifeboat, the cruiser was brought to safety. For this service, a Letter of Thanks from the RNLI Chairman was presented to Coxswain Frank Ide and the Poole crew. After nine years at Poole, Augustine Courtauld spent two years at Troon, being replaced there by a new 52ft Arun. After three further years in the Relief Fleet, she went to Arklow for the last seven years of her twenty-three-year career. She left Arklow in April 1997, and was sailed to the RNLI Depot at Poole, where she was stored for over two years, before being repainted in RVCP colours at Souter Marine, Cowes.

After service

Augustine Courtauld was sold out of service on 21 May 1999 to the Royal Volunteer Coastal Patrol, Australia. Renamed P&O Nedlloyd Strathaird (after the ship that transported her), she entered service in the Broken Bay Division as a coastguard vessel and lifeboat. She served there from 1999 to 2002, then moved to Trial Bay Division, NSW, until 2011. In May 2011 she was acquired by Melbourne Charter Services, operator of work boats in the Port of Melbourne, providing services including security and towage. She was returned to her RNLI colours, renamed Augustine Courtauld and based at Yaringa Boat Harbour, Western Port Bay, Somerville, Victoria.

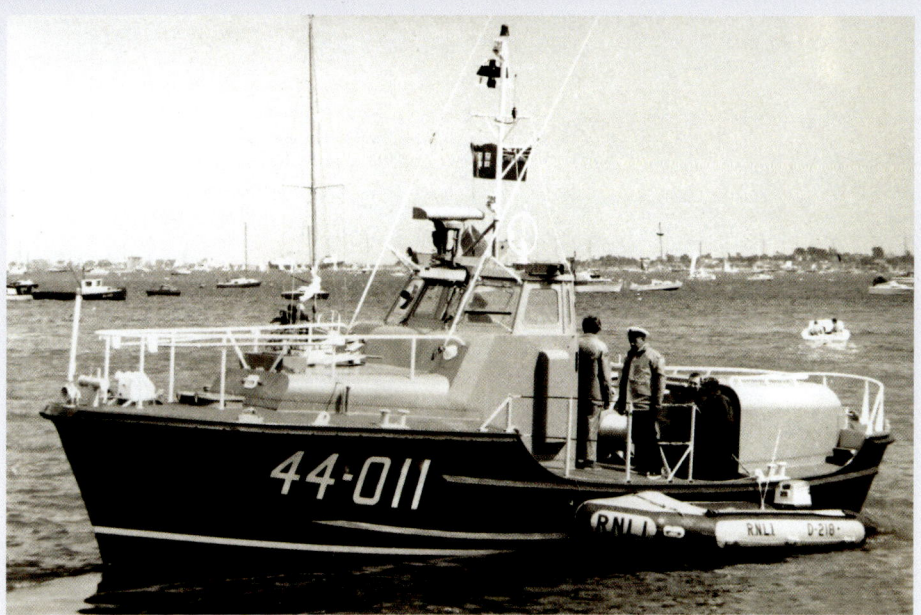

▲ 44-011 at Poole, her first station, in the mid-1970s. (Jeff Morris)

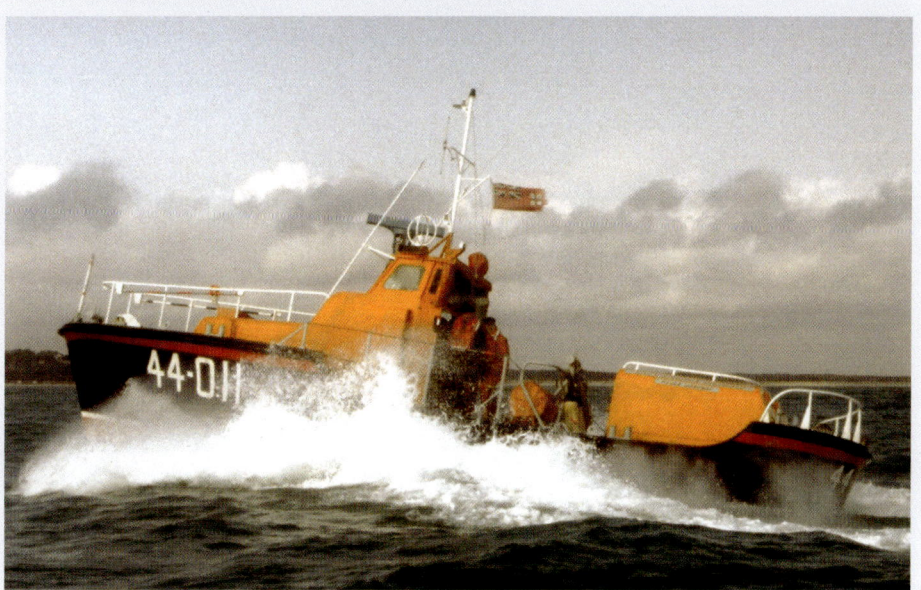

▲ 44-011 on exercise off Poole, the station she served for nine years. (By courtesy of the RNLI)

Augustine Courtauld

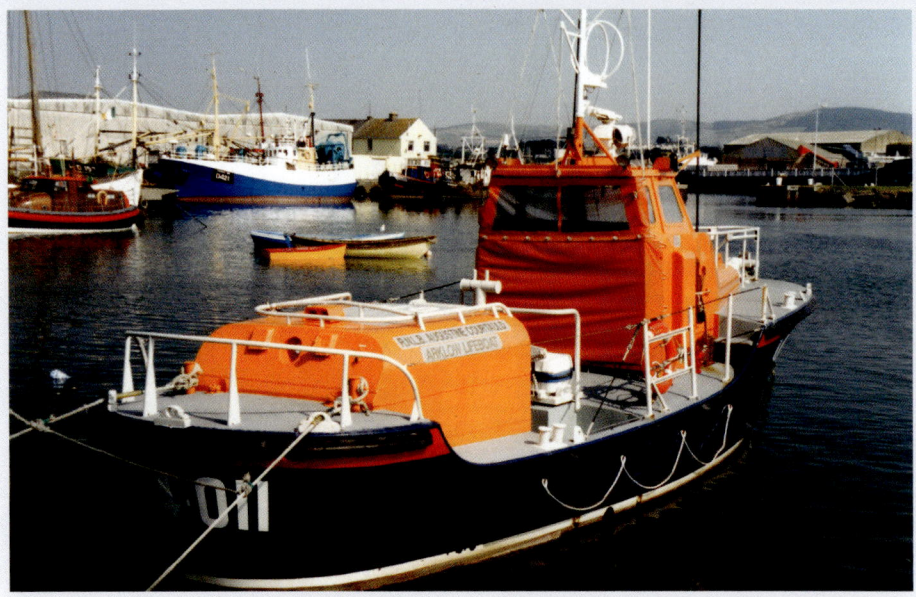

▲ 44-011 moored at Arklow, August 1995; she served the station for almost seven years. (Nicholas Leach)

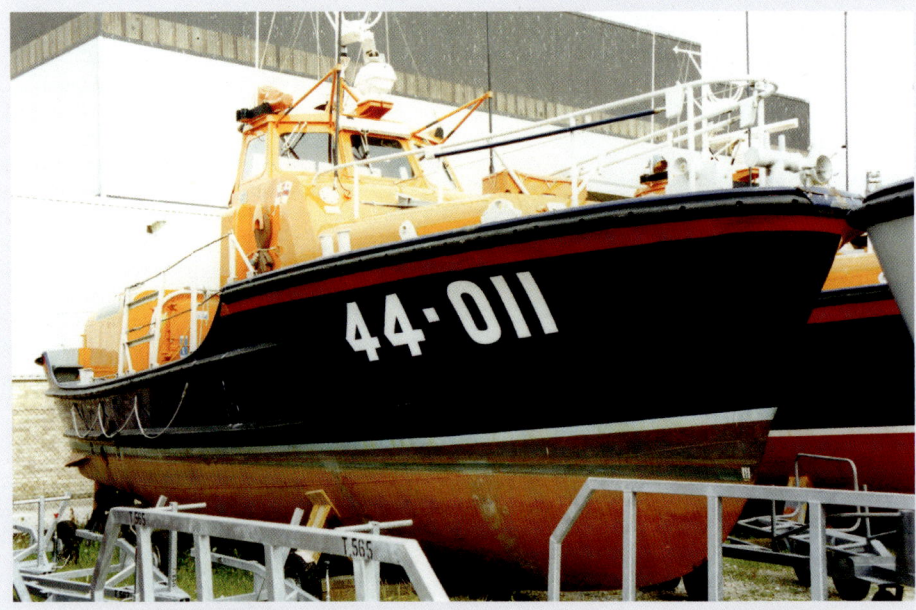

▲ 44-011 at the RNLI Depot, Poole, awaiting disposal from the RNLI fleet, July 1997. (Nicholas Leach)

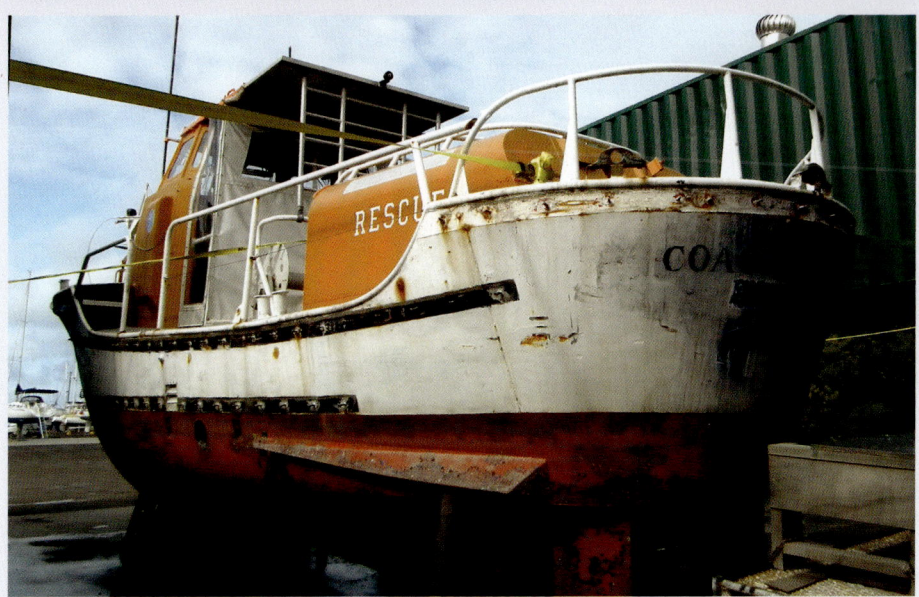

▲ 44-011 at Yaringa, Australia, shortly after being sold by the RVCP, July 2011. (Andrew Mackinnon)

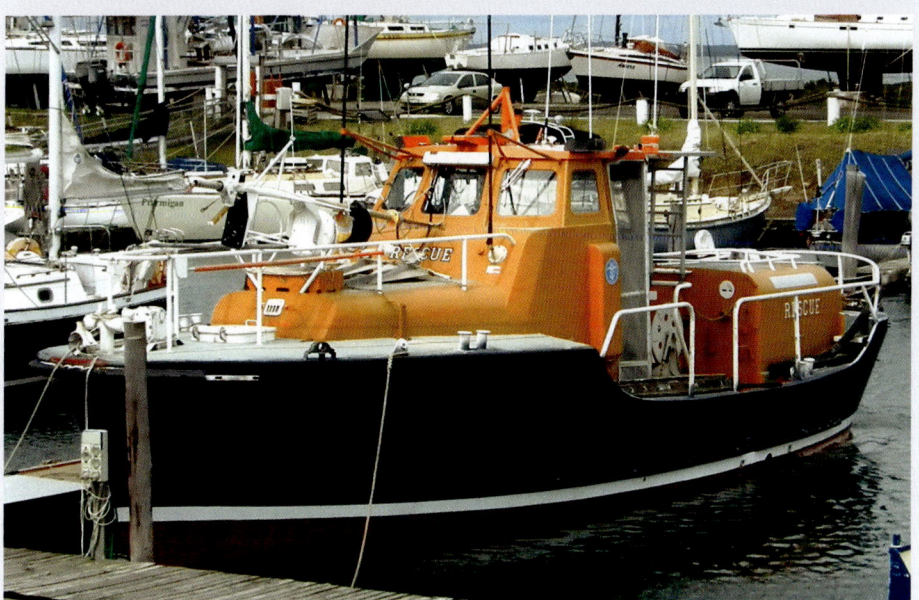

▲ 44-011 at Yaringa Marina, Western Port Bay, Australia, September 2011. (Andrew Mackinnon)

The White Rose of Yorkshire

Key data

Built 1974, Groves & Guttridge, Cowes, yard no. G&G 663

Donor Gift of Miss Gwynaeth Milburn, Harrogate

Named 21 May 1975 at Whitby by HRH Duchess of Kent, wife of the RNLI President

Cost £79,018.34

Stations Whitby 24 Nov 1974 – Dec 1988 (239/51), Invergordon 1 Apr 1989 – May 1996 (66/10), Relief May 1996 – 1997 (1/0)

Disposal Sold 15 Mar 1999 to Canadian Lifeboat Institution.

Service career

The White Rose of Yorkshire served at Whitby for fourteen years, undertaking well over 200 services. One of the most notable took place on 9 April 1988 when the 24ft yacht Cymba was swamped by heavy, breaking seas as she entered Whitby harbour, and was swept onto rocks to the west. The Whitby ILB D-260 Gwynaeth was launched followed by The White Rose of Yorkshire. The ILB picked up a man from the water but was unable to approach the casualty as conditions were beyond its limits, so the Waveney was taken in, stern first, keeping her head to sea. She gradually edged towards the casualty, despite being in danger of striking the bottom. Two approaches had to be abandoned, but on the third attempt the lifeboat got close enough for a line to be thrown across with which the lifeboat crew hauled the survivor alongside the lifeboat, then pulled him aboard. For this rescue, Coxswain/Mechanic Peter Thomson was awarded the Bronze medal, as was ILB helmsman Nicholas Botham; medal service certificates went to the other lifeboatmen involved. After Whitby, The White Rose of Yorkshire served at Invergordon for seven years and then in the Relief Fleet.

After service

The White Rose of Yorkshire was placed on the sale list on 19 August 1998 and sold out of service on 11 June 1999 to the Canadian Lifeboat Institution/Canadian Coast Guard Auxiliary. She was repainted in the CLI's livery taking part in the parade of sail for the RNLI 175th Anniversary, at Poole, in June 1999, prior to going to Canada. She was then taken to Gorleston, where she was kept until being shipped across the Atlantic via Sheerness. She was stationed at Delta Station, Roberts Bank, just south of Vancouver. Designated 1A.001, she covered the Strait of Georgia to the south of Vancouver and was later operated by the Roberts Bank Lifeboat Society. In 2008 she was retired from CLI service and sold into private ownership, being renamed White Rose of Yorkshire, and based at Canoe Pass, Ladner, British Columbia.

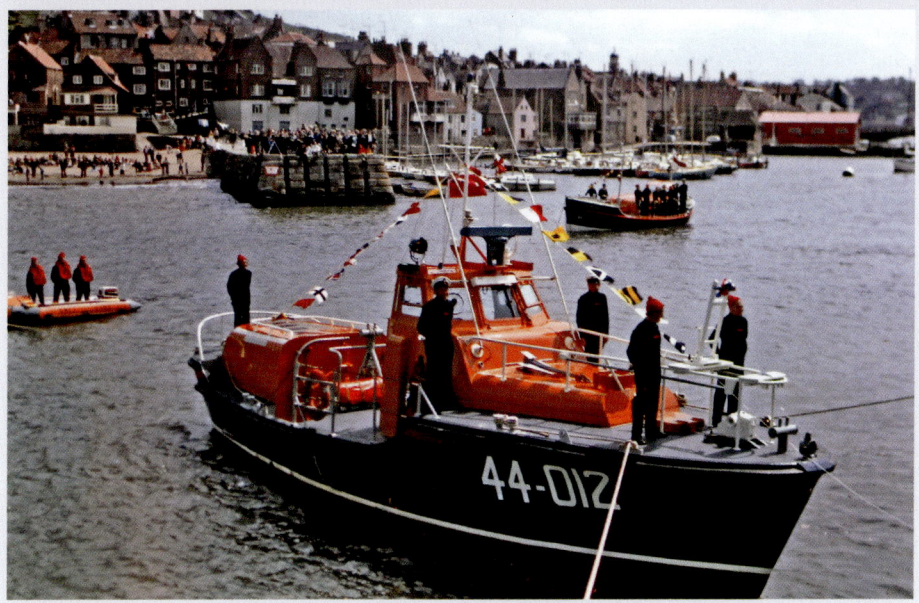

▲ 44-012 during her naming ceremony at Whitby, 21 May 1975. (Jeff Morris)

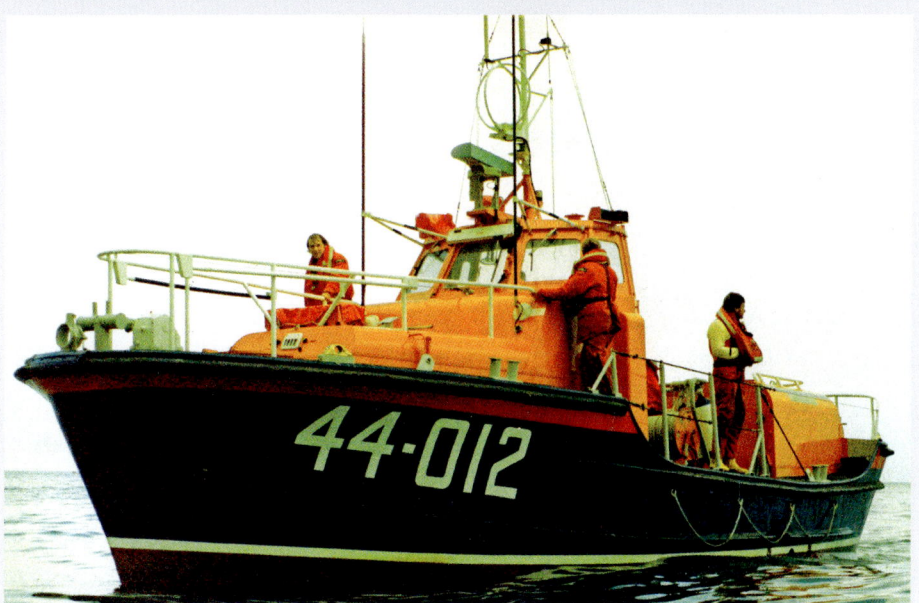

▲ 44-012 on exercise off the Yorkshire coast during her fourteen-year stint at Whitby.

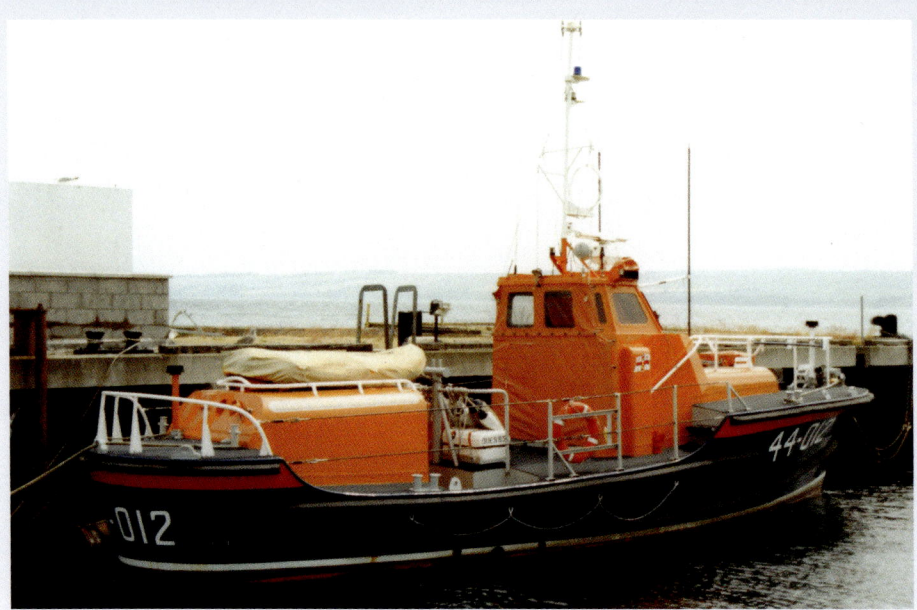

▲ 44-012 on station at Invergordon, berthed in the West Harbour, July 1995. (Nicholas Leach)

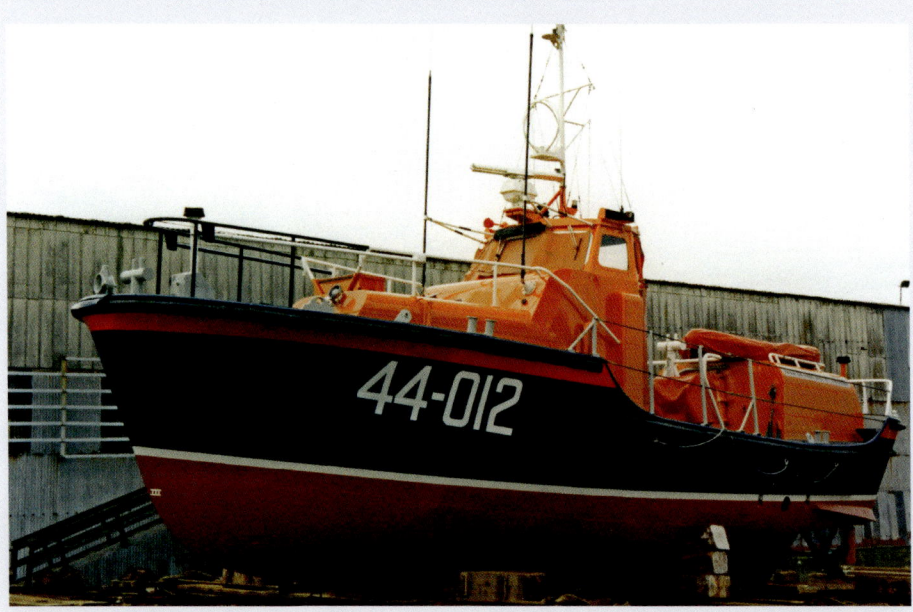

▲ 44-012 in storage at Buckie Shipyard, Buckie, August 1996, awaiting her next relief duty. (Nicholas Leach)

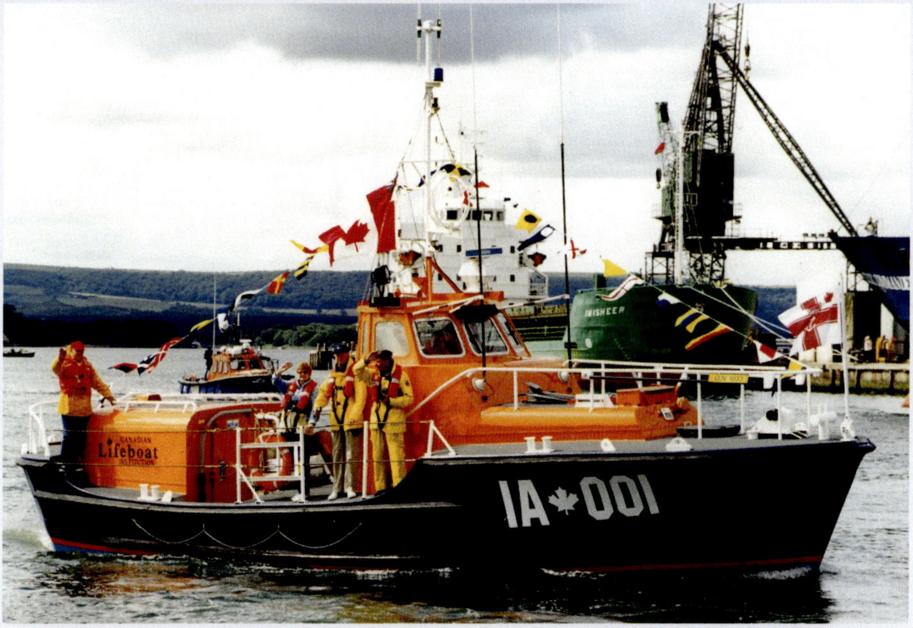

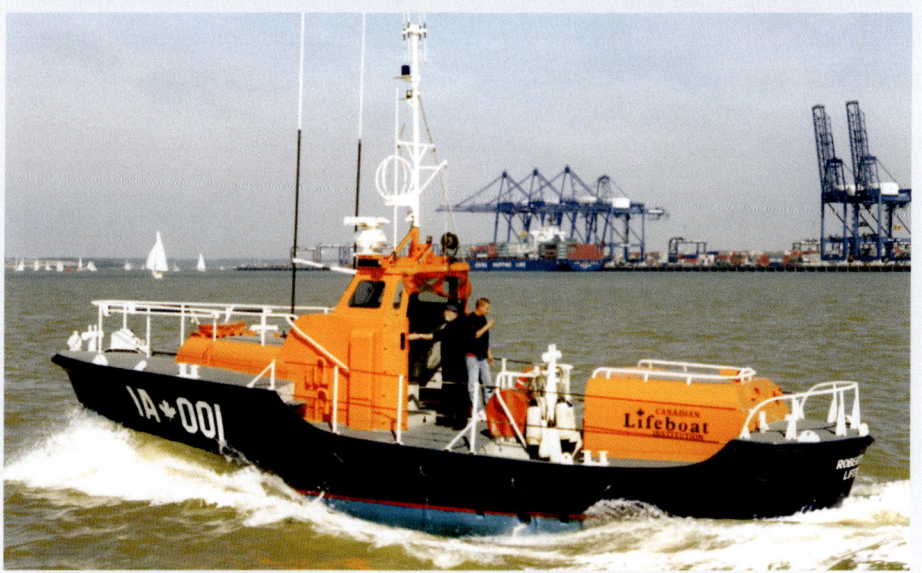

▲ 44-012 at Poole in Canadian Lifeboat Institution livery for the RNLI's 175th anniversary, June 1999.

▲ 44-012 off Harwich, August 1999, prior to being shipped to Canada. (Peter Edey)

Key data

Built 1974, Groves & Guttridge, Cowes, yard no. G&G 664

Donor Proceeds of Jersey Lifeboat Appeal.

Named 30 May 1975 at St Helier by HM Queen Elizabeth, The Queen Mother

Cost £79,049.44

Stations St Helier Feb 1975 – Dec 1989 (288/155), Relief 1989 – 1993 (20/11),
    Dunbar 1 Aug 1993 – Dec 1995 (21/0), Relief 1995 – 1997 (0/0)

Disposal Sold 13 May 1998 to Montrose Harbour Authority

Service career

Thomas James King served at the St Helier station in Jersey, and was named after one of the station's best known Coxswains, who was a Gold medal recipient. During her busy fourteen-year career in the Channel Islands, her most notable service came on 3 September 1983, when she was launched to help the yacht Cythara in gale force eight winds gusting to force nine. The lifeboat crew found the yacht in St Clement's Bay pitching heavily, so the lifeboat went alongside, and took off the three crew. As Coxswain Berry manoeuvred away, the lifeboat struck a rock, but skilful use of the engines got her clear. During a difficult return passage to station, the lifeboat again struck the bottom as she was taken though a series of rocks. For this service, in which the Waveney's steel hull proved itself, Coxswain Berry was awarded the Silver medal, with rhe Thanks Inscribed on Vellum being accorded to the rest of the crew. After leaving St Helier, Thomas James King was stationed at Dunbar for just over two years, in between spells in the Relief Fleet; her last relief duties were at Invergordon and Portree.

After service

Thomas James King was sold out of service in August 1998 to the Montrose Harbour Authority for use as a pilot boat. Renamed North Esk and based in Montrose Docks, she was repainted with a white superstructure and the wheelhouse was enclosed. In 2010 she was offered for sale for £55,000 from Montrose Harbour Commissioners, having been re-engined in 2005 with new 260hp Caterpillar diesels. She was bought in 2012 by Bay Towage & Salvage Co, Anchorline Basin, Barrow-in-Furness, and was to be taken to Barrow, via Inverness, for use as a work boat. However, in 2013 she was on the Clyde and being offered for sale through Scott Yacht Brokers Ltd, Rothesay Dock, Clydebank. In July 2013 she was bought by Ledra Ena Shipping of Cyprus and, renamed Ledra Express, was used as a work boat at the port of Limassol, Cyprus; her duties including crew transportation.

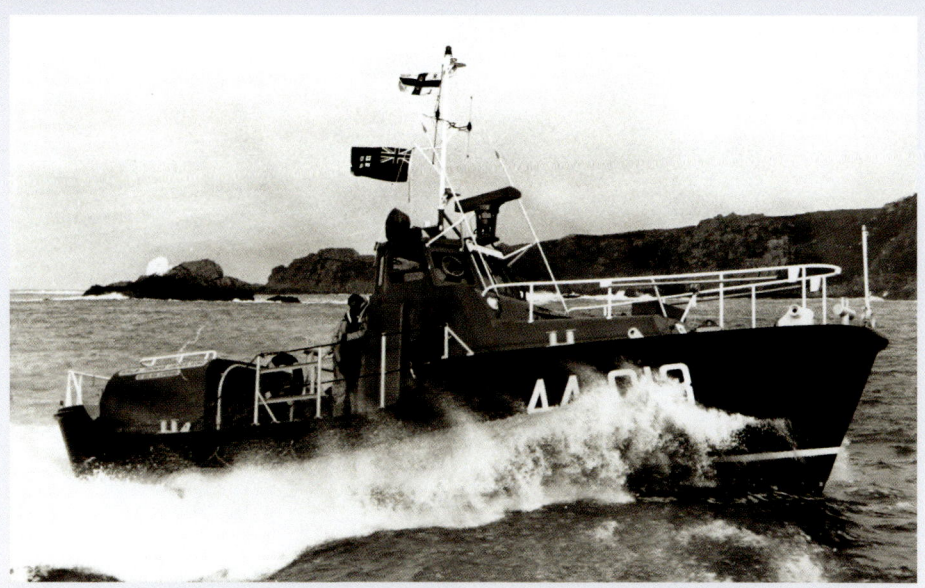

▲ 44-013 at St Helier, the station in the Channel Islands she served for more than fourteen years. (RNLI)

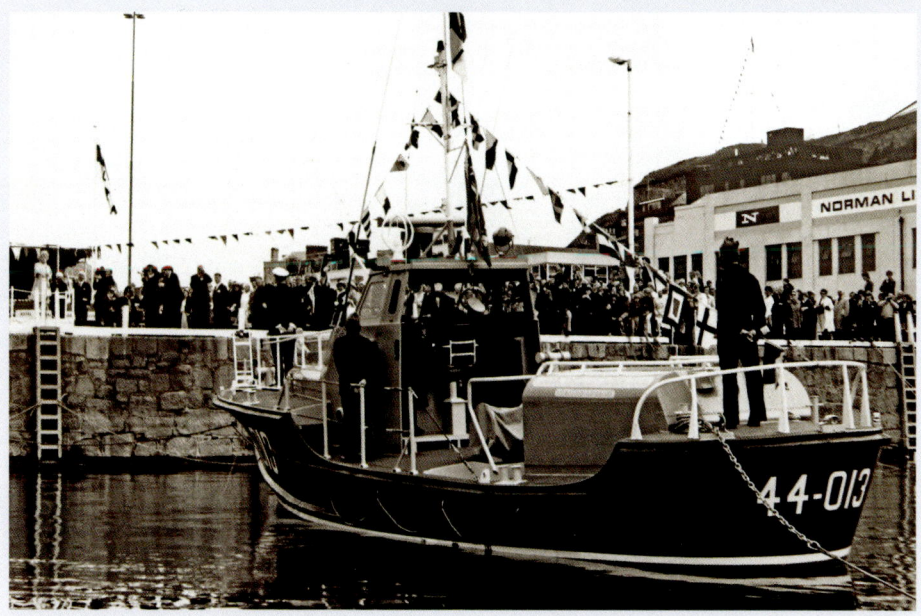

▲ 44-013 at St Helier during her naming ceremony, 30 May 1975. (By courtesy of the RNLI)

▶ 44-013 at her berth in St Helier Harbour during her time serving in the Channel Islands, August 1996.

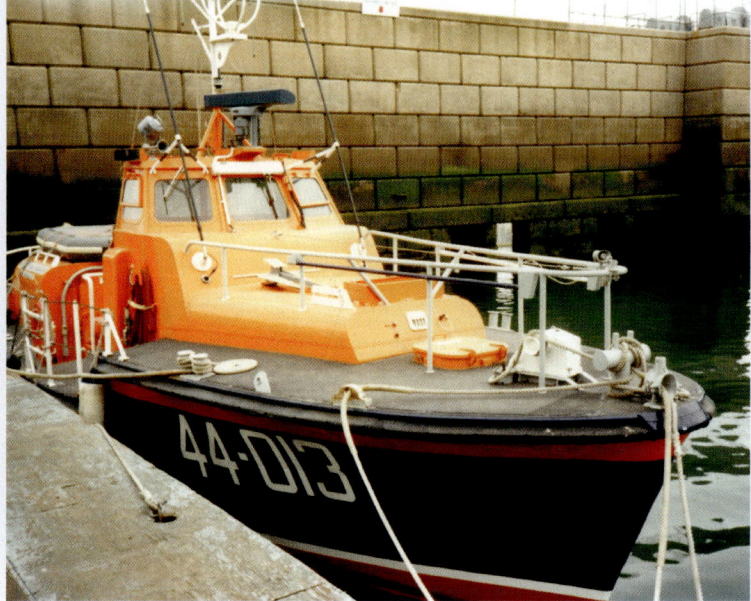

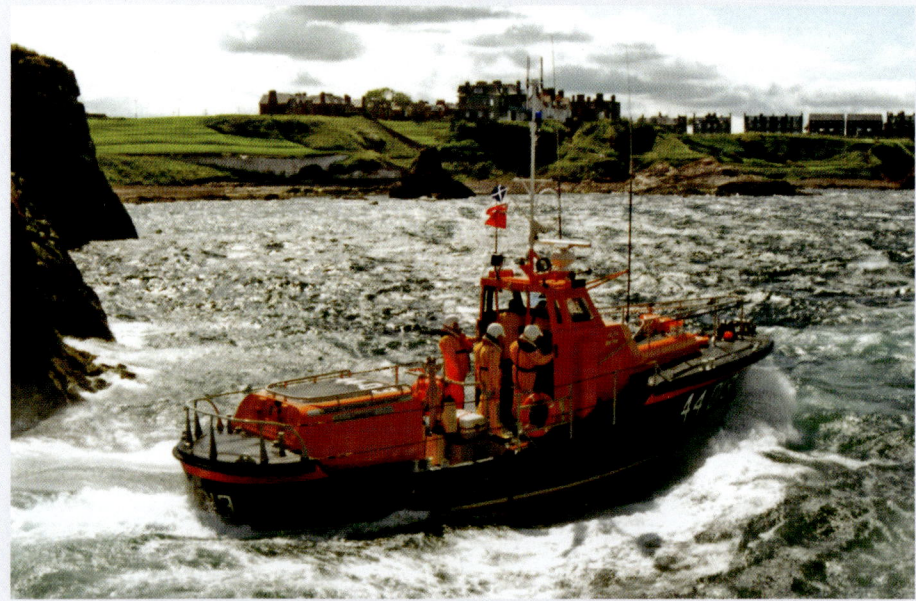

▲ 44-013 heading out of the harbour at Dunbar, July 1993. (Steve Dutton)

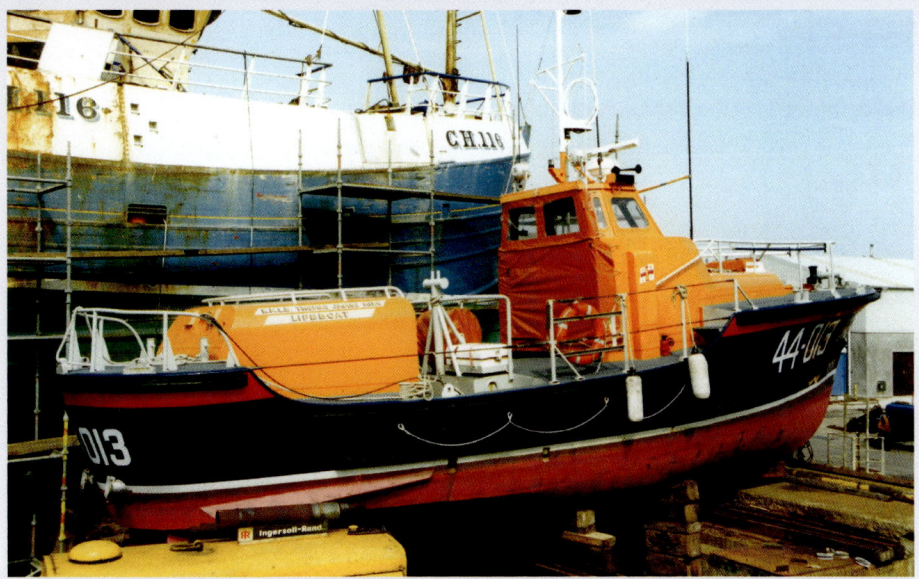

▲ 44-013 at Buckie Shipyard, Buckie, August 1997, after completing her last relief duty. (Nicholas Leach)

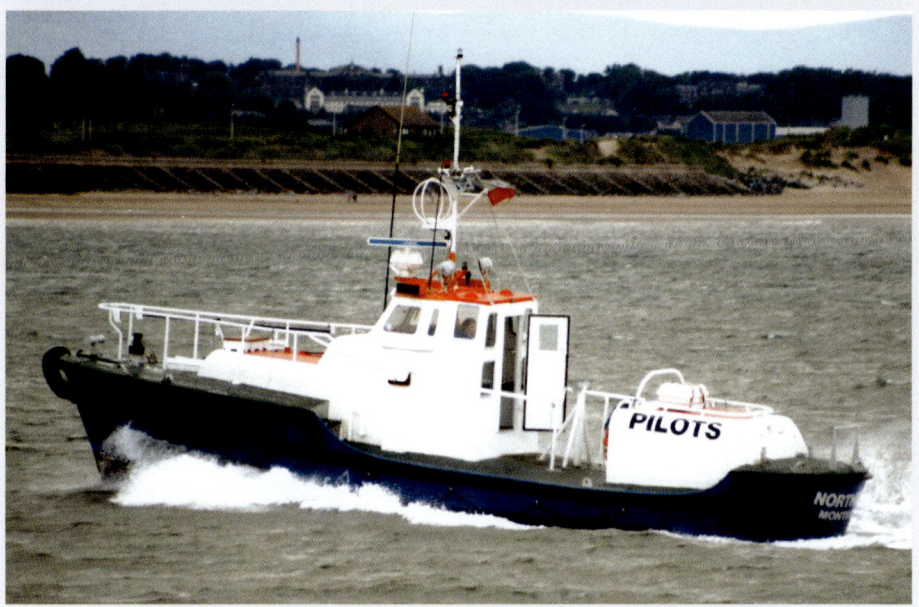

▲ 44-013 as the pilot boat North Esk returning to Montrose harbour, July 2000. (Nicholas Leach)

St Patrick

Key data

Built 1974, Groves & Guttridge, Cowes, yard no. G&G 661
Donor Proceeds of the Irish Lifeboat Appeal
Named 14 Sep 1975 at Dunmore East by Mrs Peter Barry, wife of the Minister for
  Transport and Power
Cost £79,581.98
Stations Dunmore East 19 Mar 1975 – Oct 1996 (252/83)
Disposal Sold 21 May 1999 to Royal Volunteer Coastal Patrol, Australia

Service career

St Patrick spent her entire RNLI career at Dunmore East on Ireland's south coast. Among the many notable services she carried out at Dunmore East, the most arduous took place on 9 July 1976. She was launched at 3.05am under the command of Coxswain Stephen Whittle to help the occupants of a small boat that had gone onto rocks at the foot of 100ft high cliffs with no landing place. To approach the rock, the lifeboat negotiated a very shallow channel during which the crew illuminated the scene with parachute flares and the searchlight. Coxswain Whittle slowly took the lifeboat into the Inner Channel where he could see the casualty on the rocks. Using a line thrown to him by the lifeboat crew, one survivor was pulled to safety, by which time the lifeboat was operating in less than 20ft of water and was only 20ft from the cliffs. Once the survivor had been picked up, the lifeboat had to go astern to avoid the rocks. St Patrick's crew then lost sight of the wrecked boat, and although the lifeboat was taken back in to look for the other survivor, there was no sign of either him or the boat. For this outstanding service, the Bronze medal was awarded to Coxswain/Mechanic Whittle and medal service certificates were presented to the rest of the crew.

After service

St Patrick was placed on the sale list on 14 August 1997 and sold out of service on 21 May 1999 to the Royal Volunteer Coastal Patrol, Australia. Renamed P&O Nedlloyd Strathnaver (after the ship that transported her), she entered service in the Batemans Bay Division as a coastguard vessel and lifeboat. She was later renamed P&O Nedlloyd Strathnaver Community Spirit, and was the last Waveney in service in Australia. In October 2009 she was sold to David Yule, who took her to the Mornington Peninsula, Victoria, Australia and by 2012 she was kept at Yaringa Marina, Western Port, Victoria, being used as a pleasure boat named St Patrick Strathnaver.

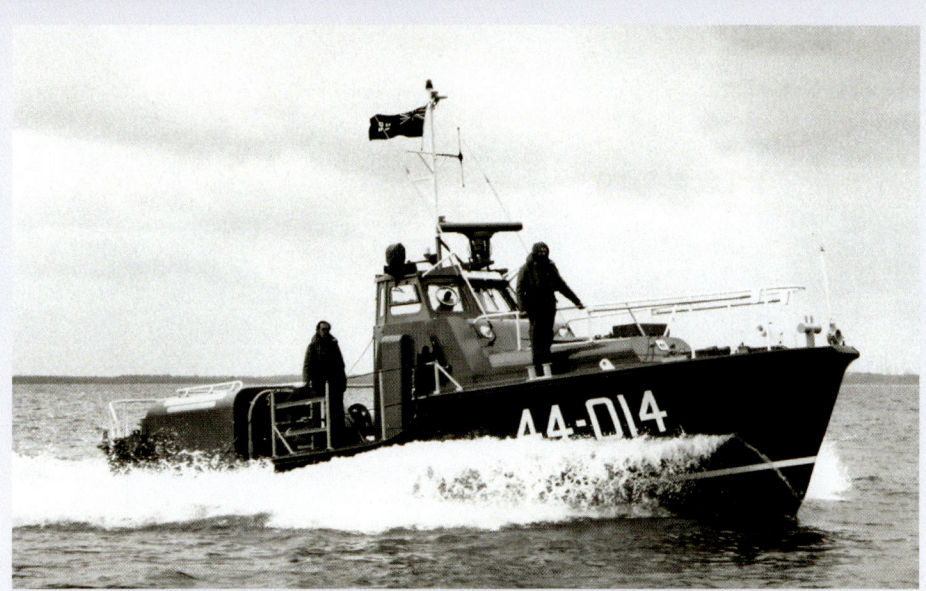

▲ 44-014 on trials soon after completion by Groves & Guttridge, Cowes. (By courtesy of the RNLI)

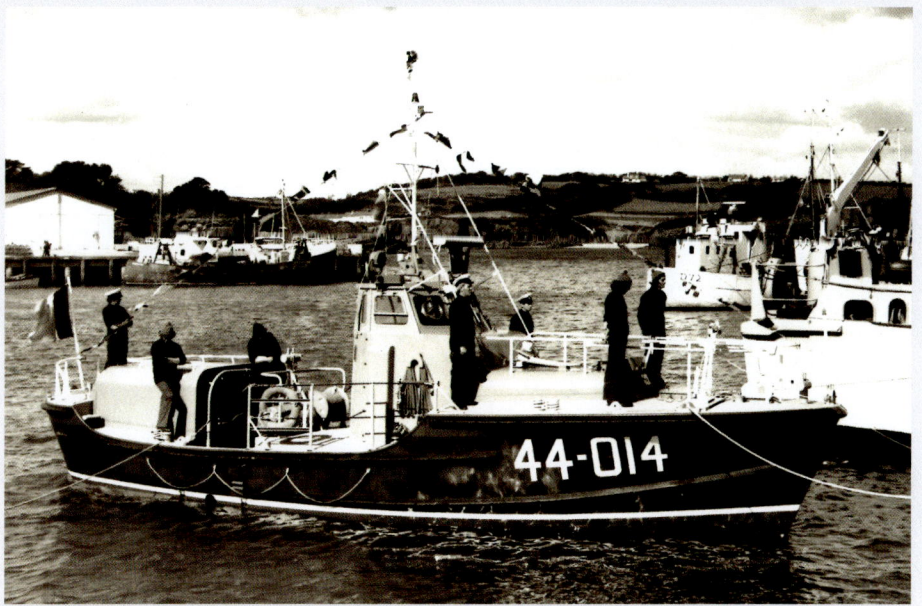

▲ 44-014 naming ceremony at Dunmore East, 14 September 1975. (By courtesy of the RNLI)

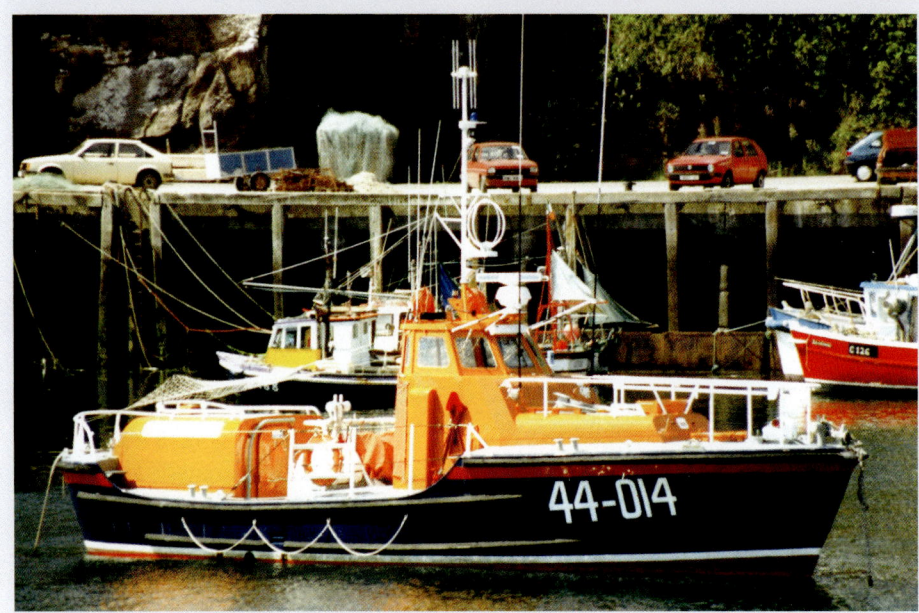

▲ 44-014 at moorings in Dunmore East Harbour, August 1995. (Nicholas Leach)

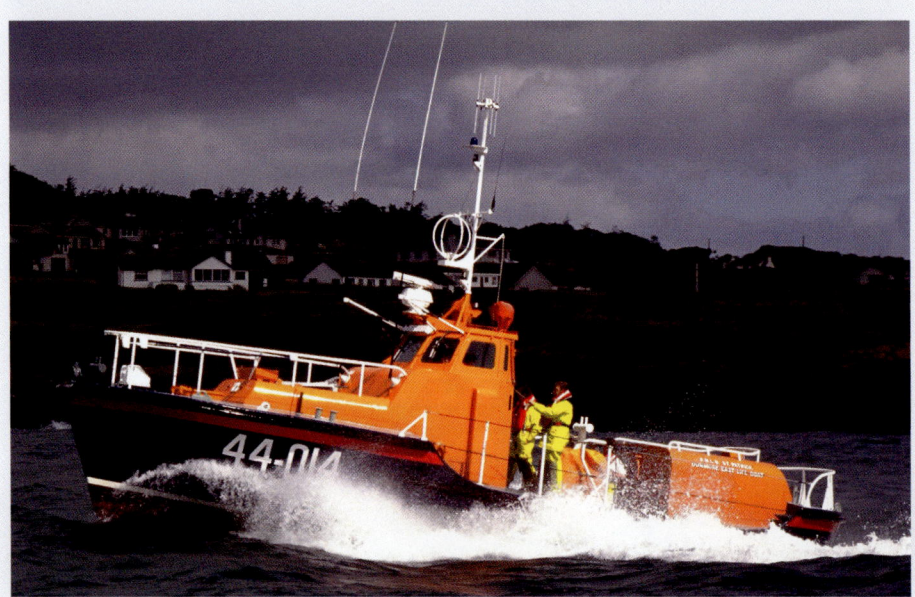

▲ 44-014 on exercise at Dumore East. (By courtesy of the RNLI)

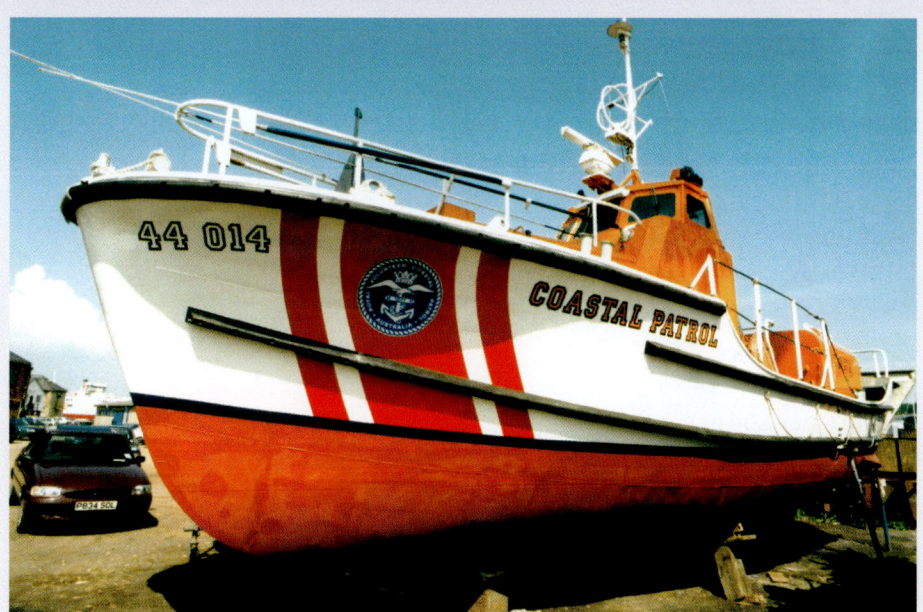

▲ 44-014 repainted in Royal Volunteer Coastal Patrol colours, Souter Shipyard, Cowes, 1999. (Peter Edey)

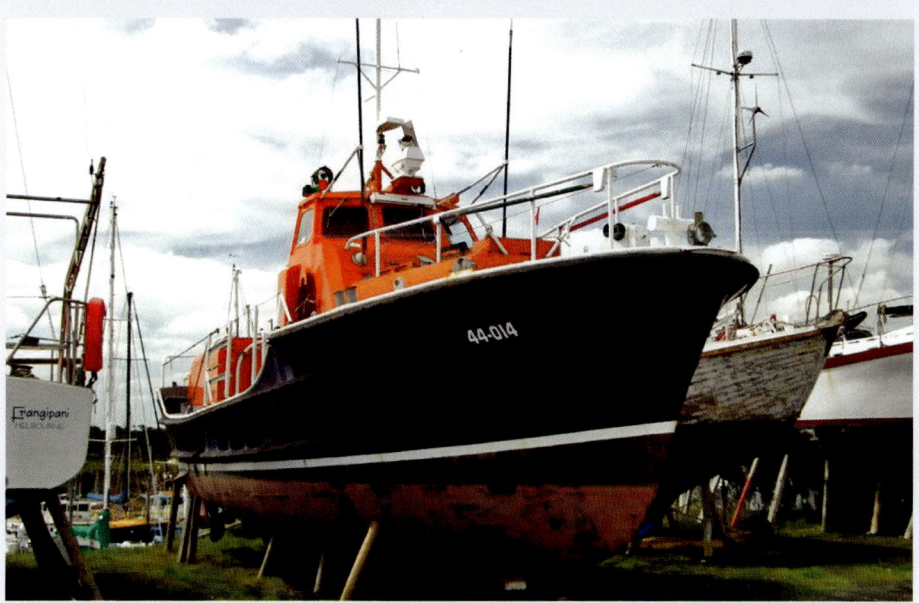

▲ 44-014 at Mornington Peninsular, Victoria, Australia in 2012, in private ownership. (Courtesy of R. Leonard)

Lady of Lancashire

Key data

Built 1974, Groves & Guttridge, Cowes, yard no. G&G 666

Donor An anonymous gift

Named 20 Jul 1976 at Fleetwood by HRH The Duke of Kent

Cost £85,967.18

Stations Fleetwood 21 Jan 1976 – 15 Oct 1989 (170/95), Dun Laoghaire 20 Mar 1990 – 10 Jan 1995 (80/4), Relief 10 Jan 1995 – 2 Nov 1996 (4/0)

Disposal Sold Nov 1996 for £55,000 to Berwick Harbour Commissioners

Service career

Lady of Lancashire gave excellent service at Fleetwood and performed 170 services, the majority of which were essentially of a routine nature. On 6 March 1989 she was involved in an extensive search for the Belgian trawler Tijl Uilenspiegel, together with six other lifeboats, as well as helicopters, aircraft, fishing vessels, merchant vessels and HMS Ribble. The trawler was lost with all hands and a large search was mounted. Lady of Lancashire launched at 11.08am to join the search, and returned to station at 8.04pm having found nothing. For their help in this extensive search, Letters of Appreciation signed by the RNLI Chief of Operations, Commodore George Cooper, were sent to the lifeboat stations involved, including Fleetwood. Following her time at the Lancashire station, she served for almost five years at Dun Laoghaire, leaving there in July 1995, being taken to Dickie's Boatyard at Bangor and then to Conwy Marina, before a passage to the RNLI Depot at Poole in May 1996 prior to being sold.

After service

Lady of Lancashire was placed on the sale list on 8 May 1996 and sold out of service in November 1996 for £55,000 to Berwick Harbour Commissioners for use as a pilot boat at Berwick-upon-Tweed. She was the first Waveney to be sold out of service, and became the third former RNLI lifeboat to be owned by the Berwick Commissioners and used for pilotage duties. She was renamed St Boisil, as the previous pilot boats had been named. The wheelhouse was enclosed and the railings were removed, but apart from these alterations she remained largely unaltered, operating as the Berwick pilot boat for longer than she had been an RNLI lifeboat.

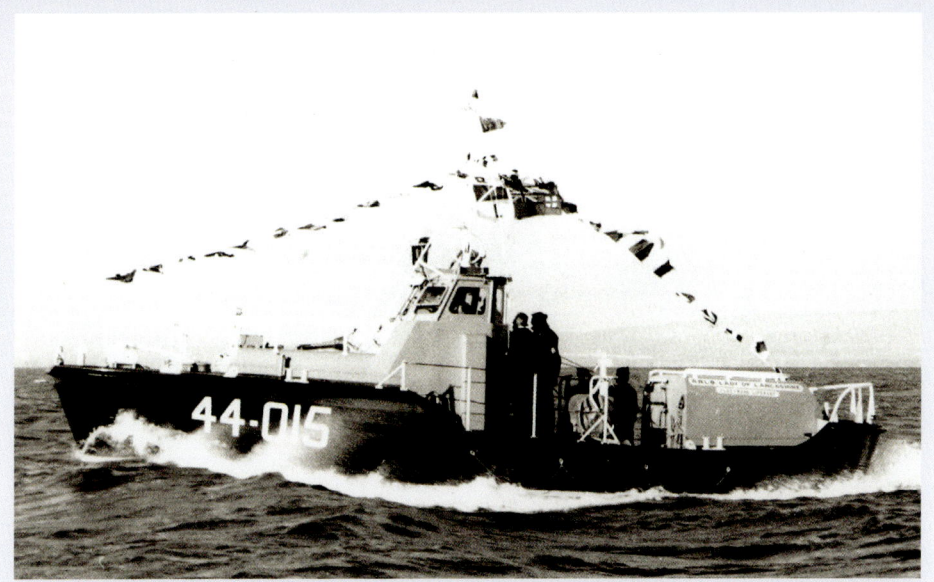

▲ 44-015 off Fleetwood after her naming ceremony, 20 July 1976. (Jeff Morris)

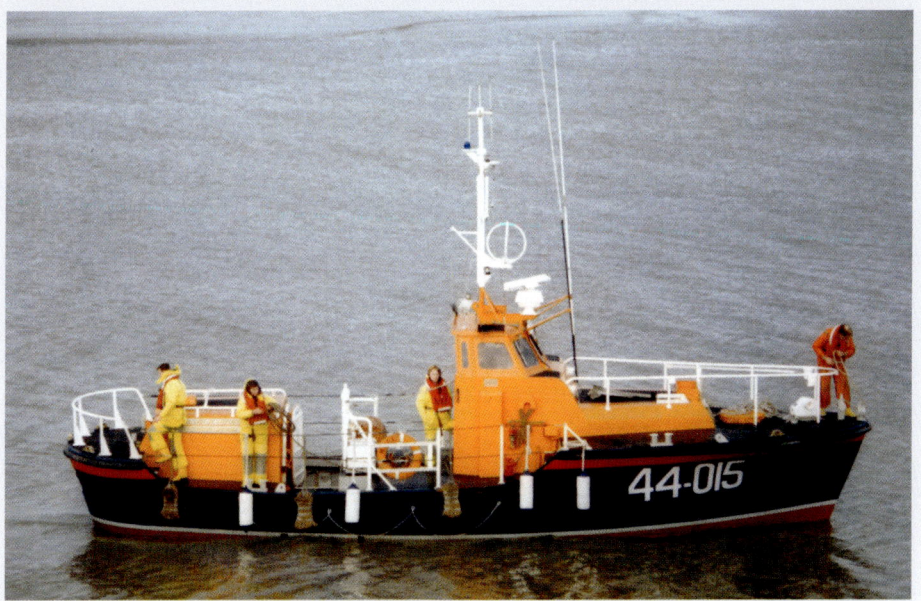

▲ 44-015 served at Fleetwood for almost fourteen years. (By courtesy of Martin Fish)

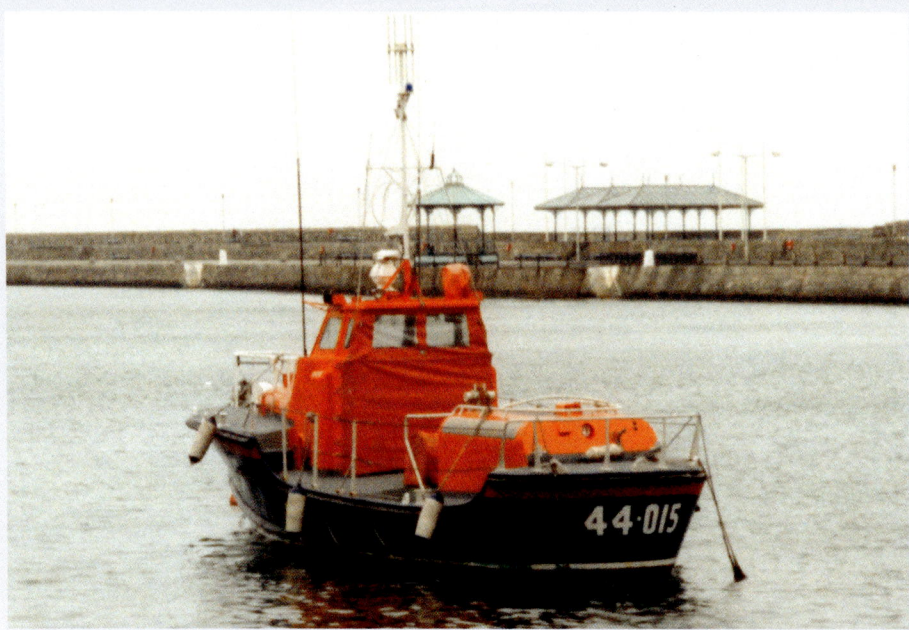

▲ 44-015 at her morings on station at Dun Laoghaire. (Supplied by Martin Fish)

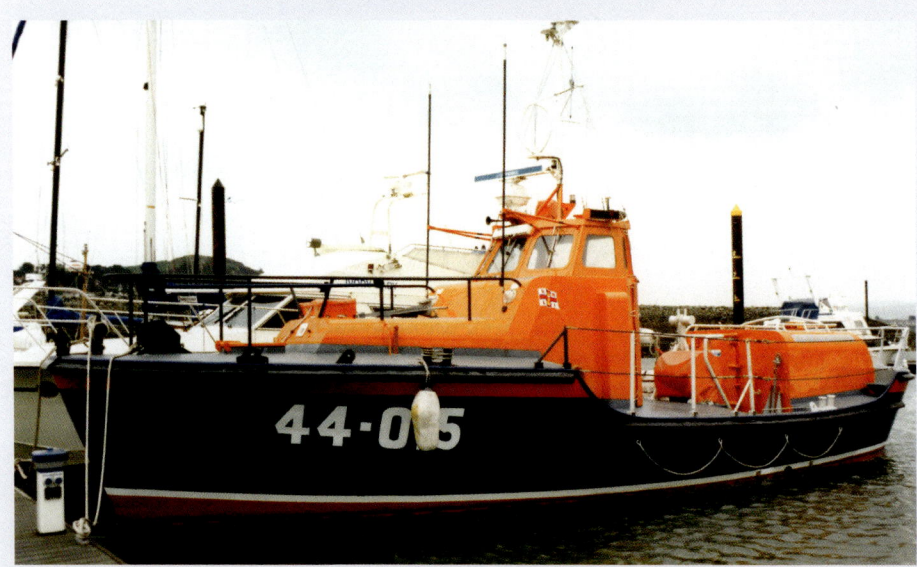

▲ 44-015 at Conwy Marina, North Wales, April 1996. (Nicholas Leach)

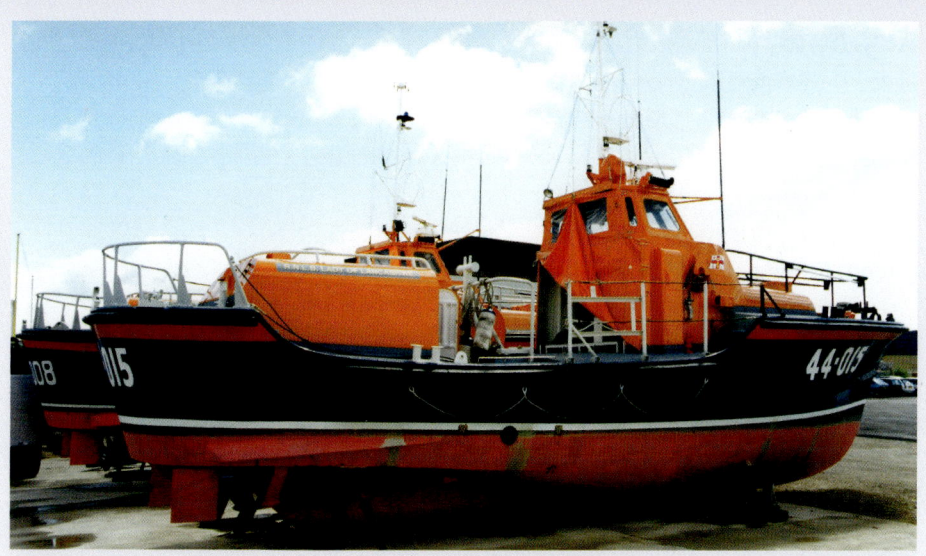

▲ 44-015 awaiing sale at the RNLI Depot, Poole, July 1996. (Nicholas Leach)

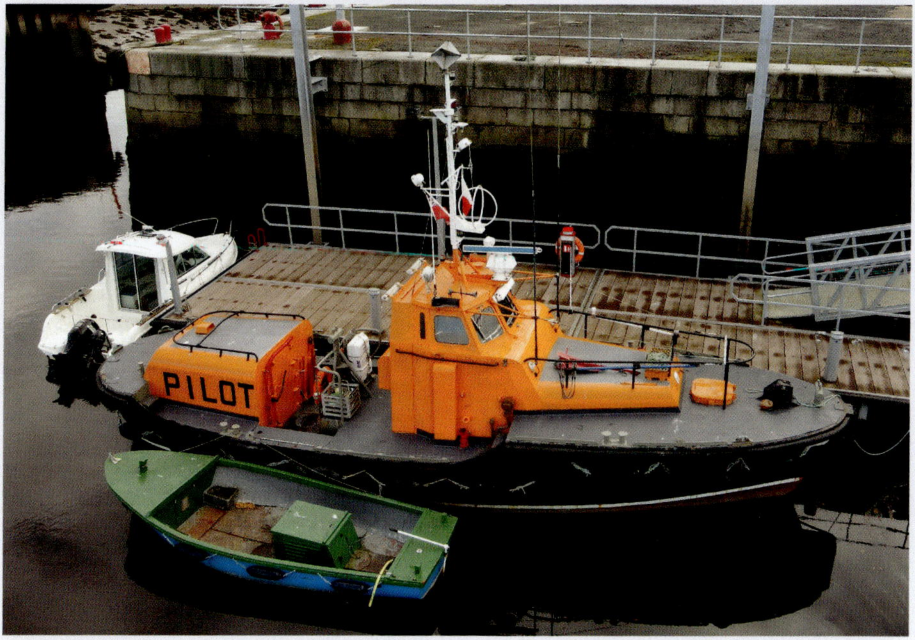

▲ 44-015 renamed St Boisil in use as a pilot boat at Berwick-upon-Tweed, October 2020. (Nicholas Leach)

Ralph and Joy Swann

Key data

Built 1976, Bideford Shipyard, North Devon, yard no. Y59

Donor Legacy of Mrs A.G. Crathorne and RNLI Funds

Named 23 Sep 1976 at Ramsgate by HRH Duchess of Kent, after a former Chairman of the RNLI, Commander Ralph Swann, and his late wife

Cost £128,524.51

Stations Ramsgate 14 July 1976 – Apr 1990 (292/199), Tobermory 6 Aug 1990 – Feb 1991 (14/2), Portree 2 May 1991 – June 1996 (60/4), Relief June 1996 – 1998 (13/1)

Disposal Sold out of service on 10 Jun 1998 to Robin Lee, Port Howard, West Falklands

Service career

Ralph and Joy Swann was stationed at Ramsgate, where she covered the Goodwin Sands, and undertook almost 300 rescues, including a demanding one on 17 April 1981 when she launched to the yacht Mersea Rival, which was aground on the Brake Sands in heavy seas with winds gusting to force nine. The yacht was almost under water by the time the lifeboat arrived on scene, and the yacht's eight crew had taken to the liferaft. Coxswain Ron Cannon brought the lifeboat alongside the raft in heavy breaking seas to rescue the eight people, then headed for Ramsgate. For this fine service a Letter of Appreciation, signed by the RNLI Director Rear Admiral W.J. Graham, was sent to Coxswain Cannon and the lifeboat crew. After being replaced by a 47ft Tyne at Ramsgate, Ralph and Joy Swann served at two newly established stations on the west coast of Scotland, Tobermory and Portree, spending more than five years at the latter, before a brief stint in the Relief Fleet, relieving at Dun Laoghaire and Achill.

After service

Ralph and Joy Swann was placed on the sale list on 24 February 1998 and sold out of service in July 1998 to Robin Lee, of Port Howard Lodge, Falkland Islands. She was shipped from Poole to the Falklands and arrived at Port Stanley in October 1998. She was then sailed to Port Howard, on West Falkland, a ten-hour journey, where her new owner operated a Tourist Lodge and sheep farm. She was renamed West Swann after West Swan Island in the Falkland Sound, but retained a double 'n' in Swann to commemorate her old name. During the season, she was used to take tourists on trips to see penguins, dolphins and other wildlife on the smaller islands. In January 2000 Mr Lee started suffering heart problems, and was flown to the UK for treatment, but sadly on 9 May he died of a heart attack. West Swann remained at Port Howard, and was operated by Myles Lee, Mr Lee's eldest son, but has since deteriorated.

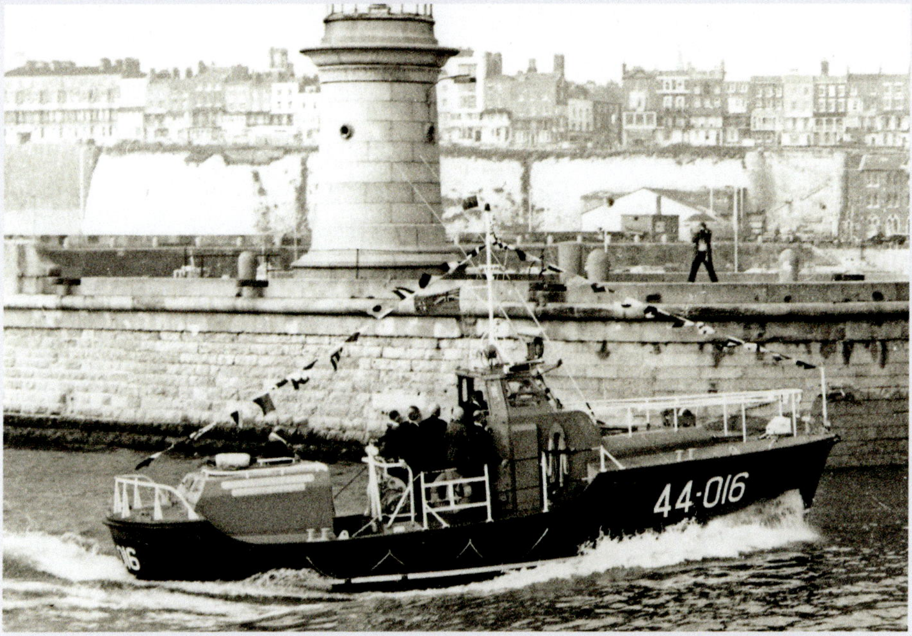

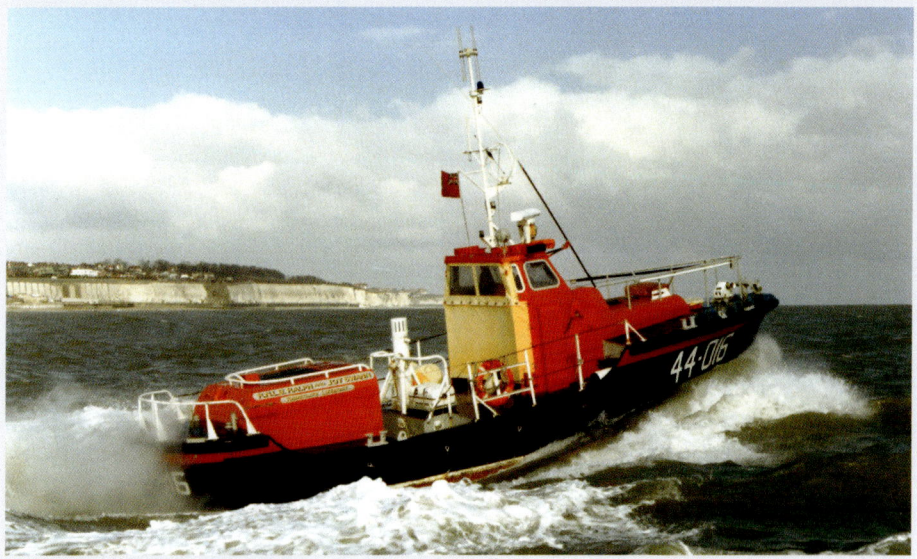

▲ 44-016 returns to Ramsgate Harbour after her naming ceremony, September 1976. (Jeff Morris)

▲ 44-016 on exercise off Ramsgate, the station she served for fourteen years, 1988. (Ray Noble)

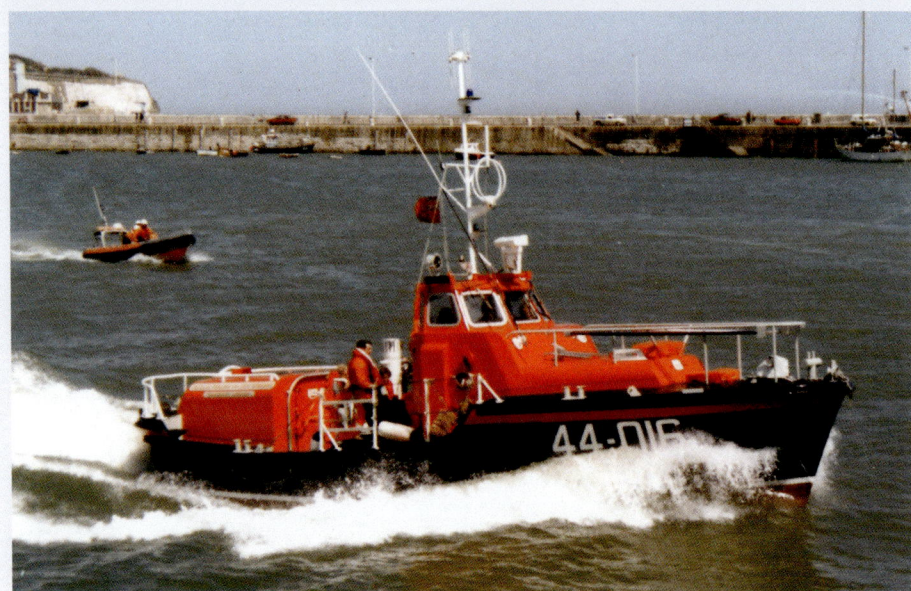

▲ 44-016 heading out of Ramsgate harbour, escorted by Atlantic 21 B-558, May 1986. (Nicholas Leach)

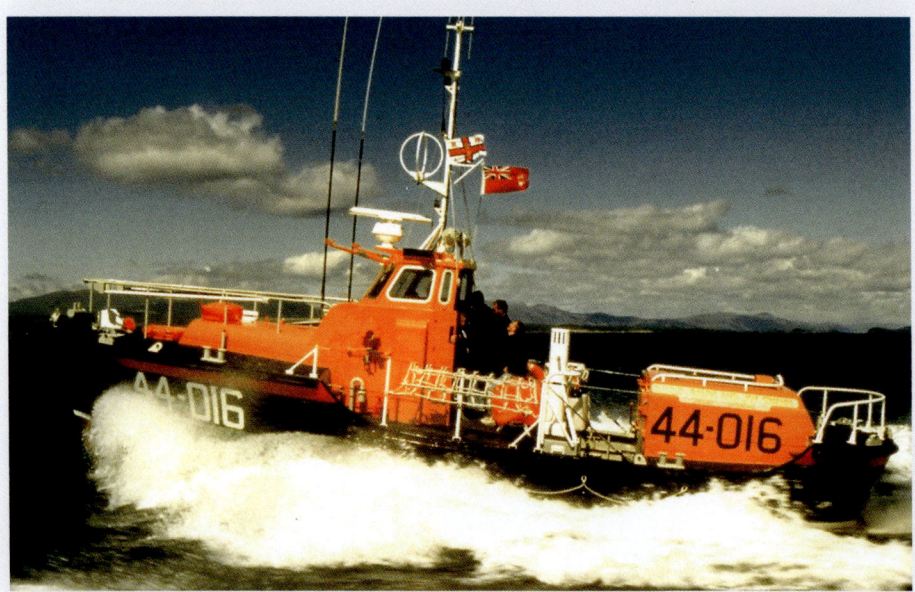

▲ 44-016 arriving on station at Tobermory in the Western Isles, May 1990. She reopened the station, from which the last lifeboat had been withdrawn in 1947. (RNLI)

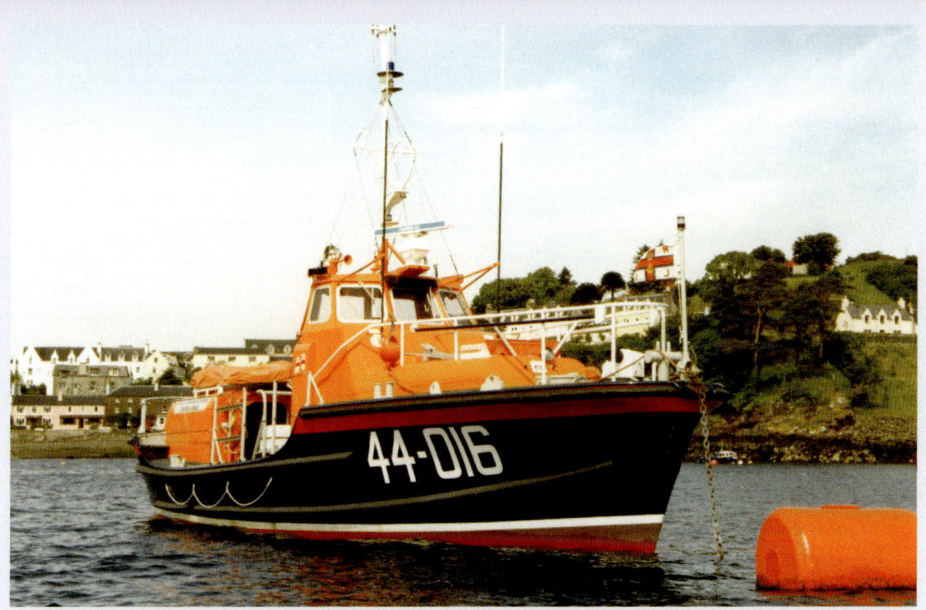

▲ 44-016 at her mooring in Portree harbour, July 1995. (Nicholas Leach)

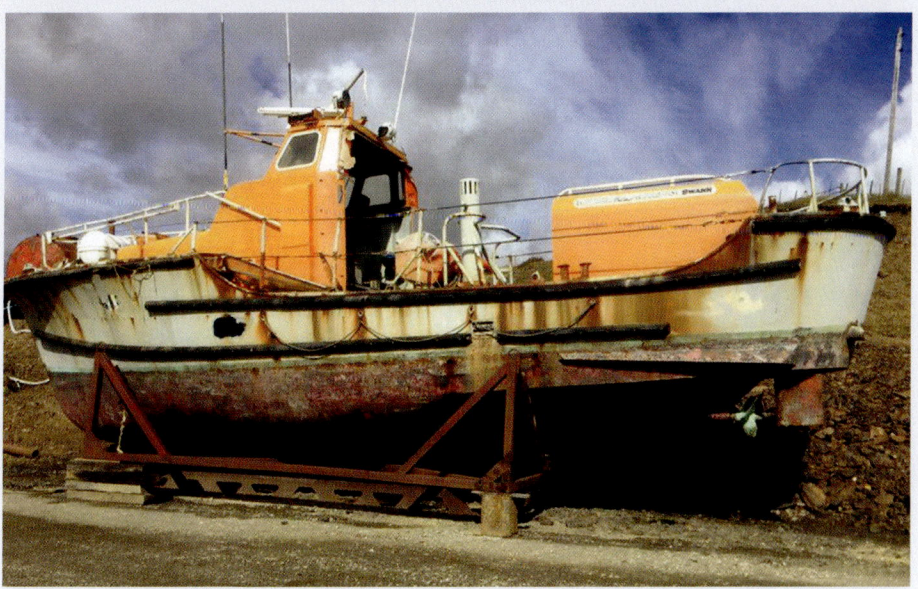

▲ 44-016, renamed West Swann, out of the water in the Falkland Islands, where she has been used as a ferry taking people and freight across Falkland Sound to Port San Carlos on East Falkland.

Key data

Built 1976, Bideford Shipyard, North Devon, yard no. Y60

Donor Various legacies plus local appeal; appropriated to the Wavy Line Grocers' Association

Named Never formally named The Nelsons of Donaghadee; named Wavy Line at a ceremony on 3 September 1980 at St Katharine Dock, London, by Mrs Barbara Laird, wife of a Wavy Line grocer from Hartley Wintney

Cost £174,688.22

Stations Donaghadee Oct 1976 – July 1977 (1/0), Relief 1978 – 1990 (111/51), Sunderland 17 Apr 1990 – 28 Mar 1997 (113/20), Relief 28 Mar 1997 – 6 Mar 1998 (0/0)

Disposal Sold 11 Nov 1997 to Mana Volunteer Coastguard, New Zealand

Service career

The Nelsons of Donaghadee was built in 1976 for Donaghadee but spent less than a year at the station due to engine problems which required her to be re-engined, after which she was reallocated to the Relief Fleet and renamed Wavy Line. When in the Relief Fleet, she carried out rescues at many different stations, including a notable one on 25 March 1983 when she was on duty at Eyemouth. She was launched to the trawler Hatcliffe, of Grimsby, which had broken down in very rough seas and winds gusting to force nine. The lifeboat rigged a tow line, but conditions were so bad that it was not possible to enter St Abbs Harbour or Berwick, where an extremely heavy swell had built up at the harbour entrance, so the lifeboat and casualty made for Burnmouth. For this service a Framed Letter of Thanks signed by the RNLI Chairman, The Duke of Atholl, was presented to Coxswain Alexander Dougal and the crew.

After service

Wavy Line was placed on the sale list on 25 April 1997 and sold out of service on 7 March 1998 to the Royal New Zealand Coastguard Federation for search and rescue based at Mana Island, near Wellington. She was shipped out from Tilbury free of charge by P&O Nedlloyd on Pegasus Bay, the first of six Waveneys to go to New Zealand. She arrived in Wellington on 30 April 1998, and was sent to Mana Marina in Porirua Harbour. The boat was funded by the Lottery Grants Board and Porirua Licensing Trust, and renamed Nicholson Rescue. In August 1999 Nicholson went into receivership so a new sponsorship deal in April 2000 saw the boat renamed Trust Porirua Rescue. In 2010 she was sold by the Coastguard and renamed Toucan in private hands, being sold again in March 2015 to Maritime Specialist Services, who removed her aft cabin, extended the wheelhouse and used her for towing, salvage and crew transport work.

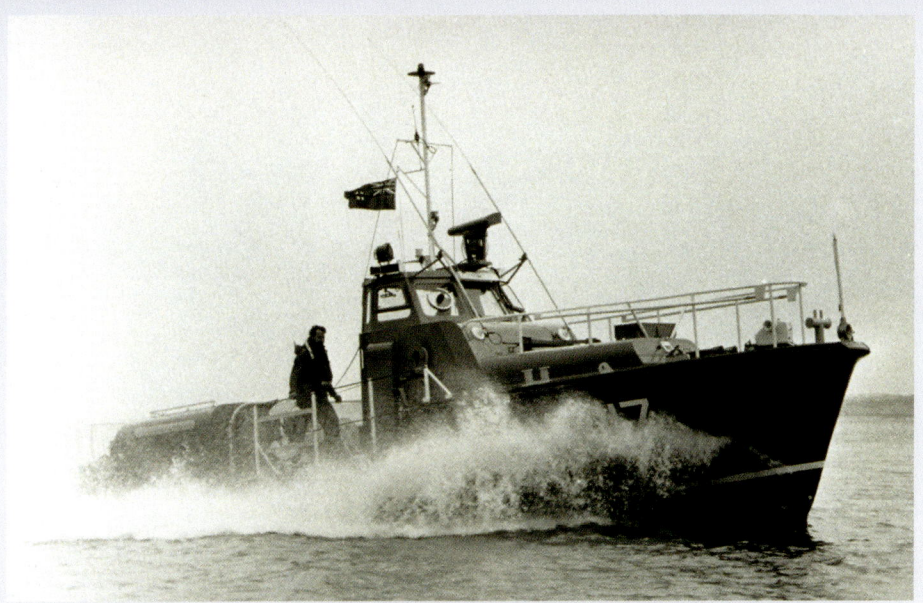

▲ 44-017 on trials in 1976, prior to going to Donaghadee. (By courtesy of the RNLI)

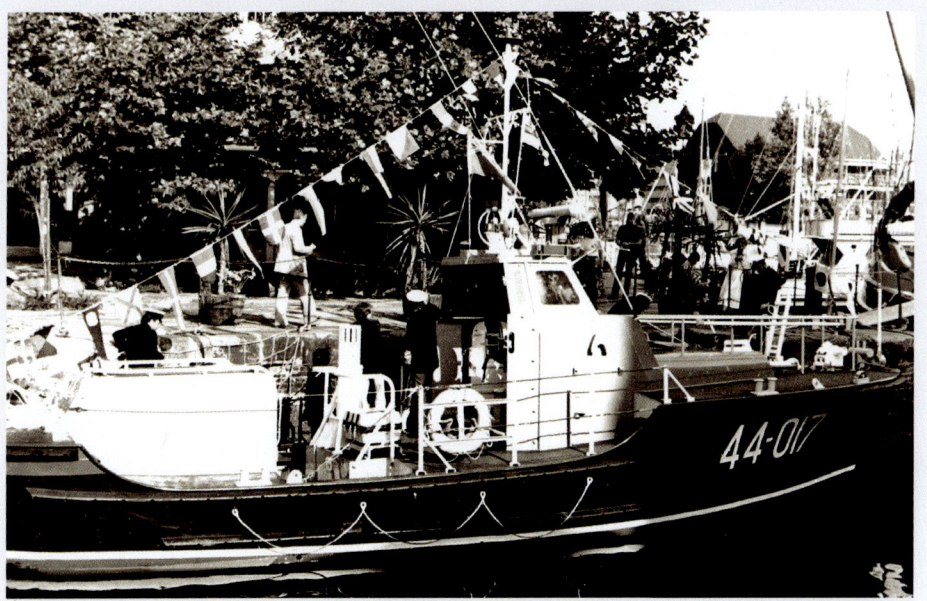

▲ 44-017 naming ceremony of Wavy Line at St Katharine Docks, London, 3 September 1980. (Jeff Morris)

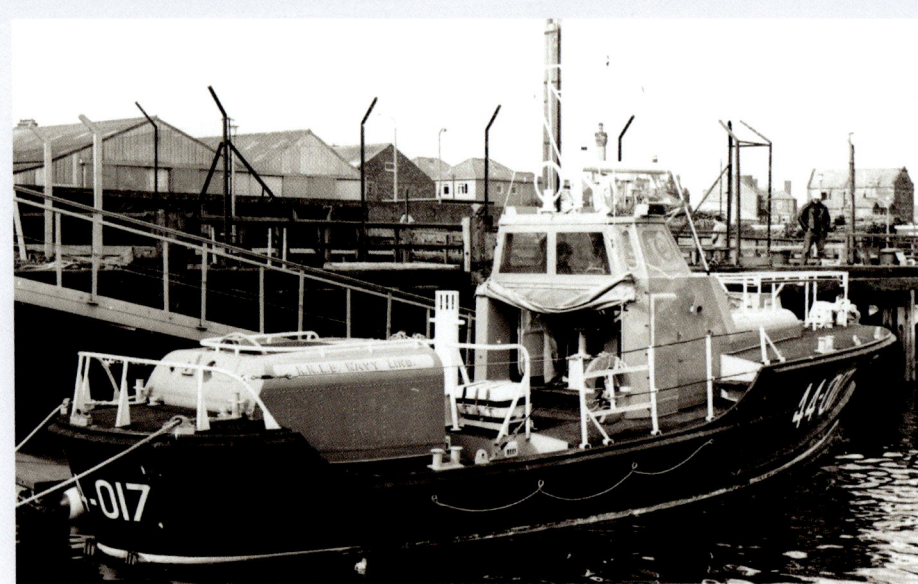

▲ 44-017 on relief duty at Blyth, standing in during the naming ceremony of Blyth's own Waveney, The William and Jane (44-022), September 1983. (Jeff Morris)

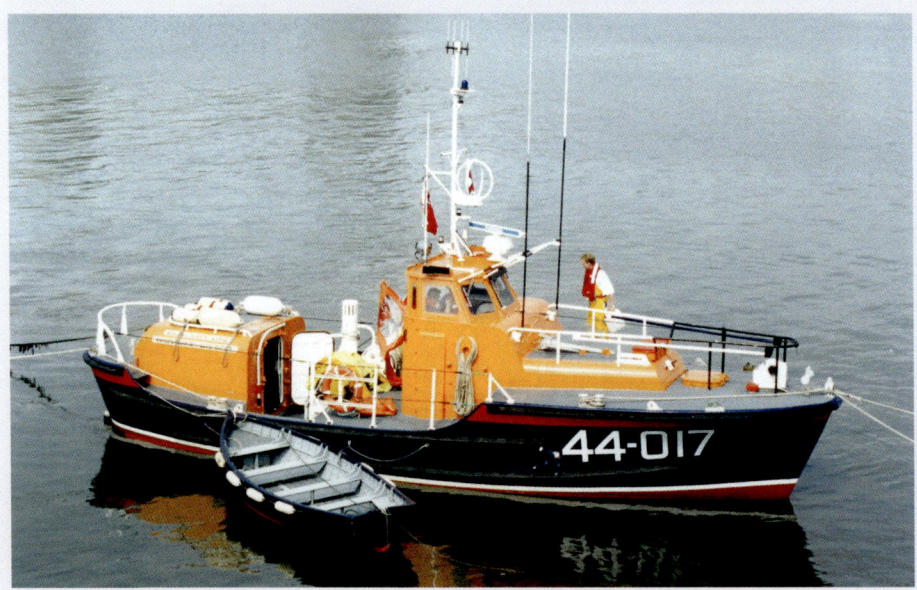

▲ 44-017 at Sunderland on her moorings following exercise, July 1994. (Nicholas Leach)

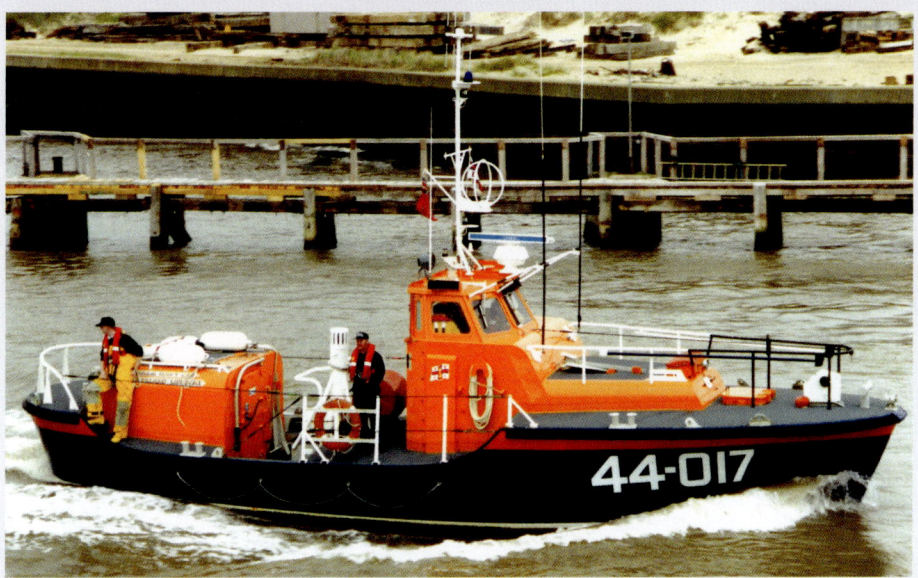

▲ 44-017 leaving Gorleston on passage to the RNLI Depot, Poole, April 1997. (Gary Markham)

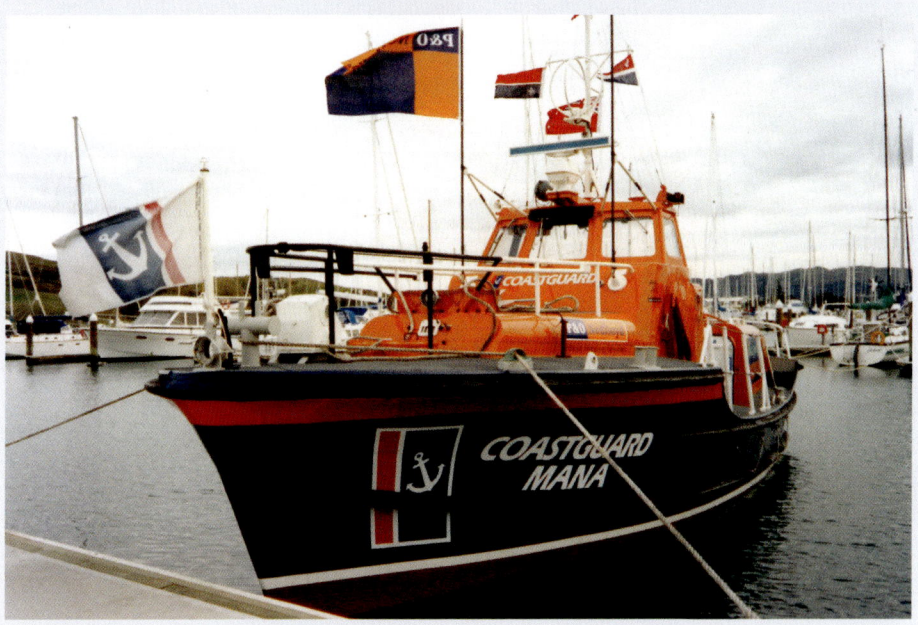

▲ 44-017 on her renaming day, when she was christened Nicholson Recsue, 21 May 1998. (V.H. Young)

The Scout

Key data

Built 1977, Bideford Shipyard, North Devon, yard no. Y61
Donor The Scout Association
Named 14 Jul 1977 at Harbour Terrace, Hartlepool, by HM Queen Elizabeth
Cost £129,079.86
Stations Hartlepool 17 Feb 1977 – July 1997 (250/10)
Disposal Sold 1997 to ADES, the Uruguayan lifeboat service

Service career

The Scout served at Hartlepool for twenty years, gaining an outstanding record of service, with her capsize on 28 February 1993 on service to the tanker Freja Svea being the only instance a Waveney capsized on service in the British Isles or Ireland. She was also involved in a number of other fine rescues, with one undertaken in the early hours of 10 November 1985 being particularly notable. After the Dutch motor coaster Anne went aground on the Long Scar rocks near Hartlepool in severe gale force nine winds gusting to force eleven, with very high seas breaking across her, The Scout went to her aid. She stood by awaiting a tug but the tug had to turn back due to the weather so the lifeboat was manoeuvred in to help. In the lee of the rocks, the waves moderated, but when the lifeboat was taken alongside a heavy sea pushed her away. A second attempt was successful, and two men were taken off before another large sea swept the lifeboat's bow off and pushed her starboard quarter against the coaster's stern. The collision slightly damaged the lifeboat's after cabin housing, but the coxswain made another run, enabling two more of the coaster's crew to be taken off. The lifeboat then stood off with the four seamen aboard. After half an hour, with the tide falling, the coaster's captain was out of immediate danger and the lifeboat headed back to Hartlepool where the men were landed at 3.06am. For this service, the Bronze medal was awarded to Coxswain Robbie Maiden and medal service certificates were presented to the rest of the crew.

After service

The Scout was placed on the sale list on 24 July 1997 and sold out of service later in 1997 to ADES, the Uruguay lifeboat service, for service at Base No1 Puerto del Buceo, a suburb of the capital, Montevideo. Transported on a container ship from Tilbury to South America, she was renamed ADES 16 14-016 in Uruguay. In 2015 she was sold by ADES and was used as a work boat at Puerto del Buceo, with her aft cabin removed and wheelhouse extended. In 2021-22 she was under renovation at Astillero Rosendo shipyard, Puerto del Buceo

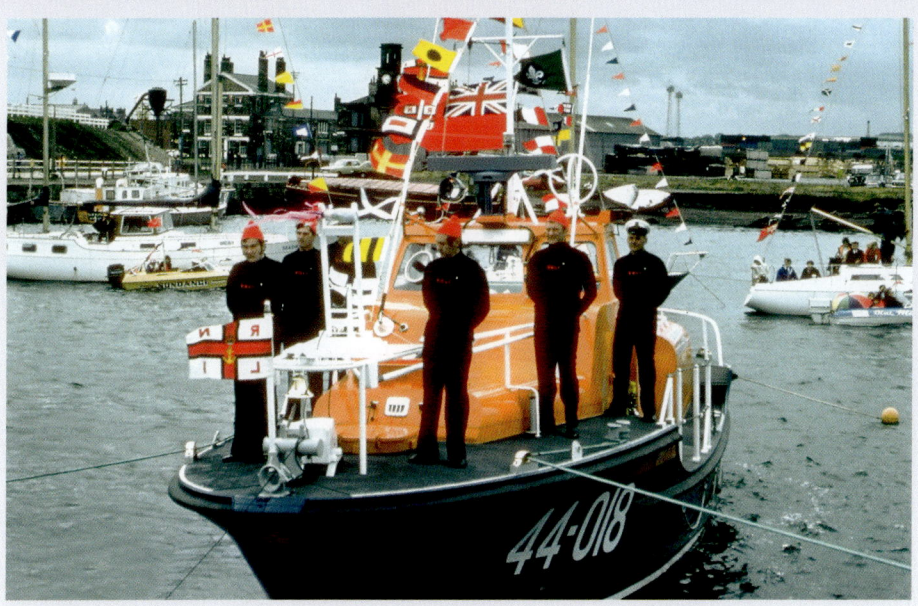

▲ 44-018 at Hartlepool during her naming ceremony, 14 July 1977. (By courtesy of the RNLI)

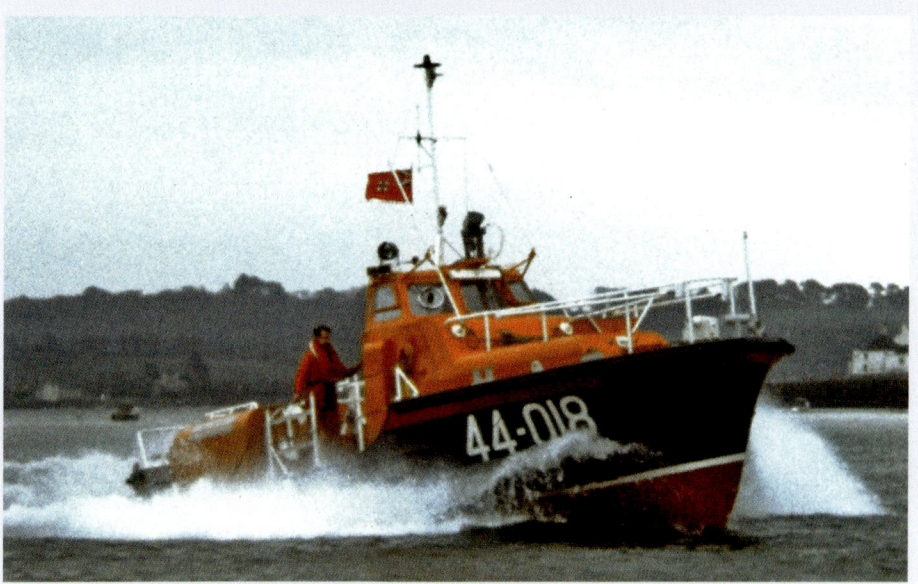

▲ 44-018 heading out of Hartlepool on exercise. (By courtesy of the RNLI)

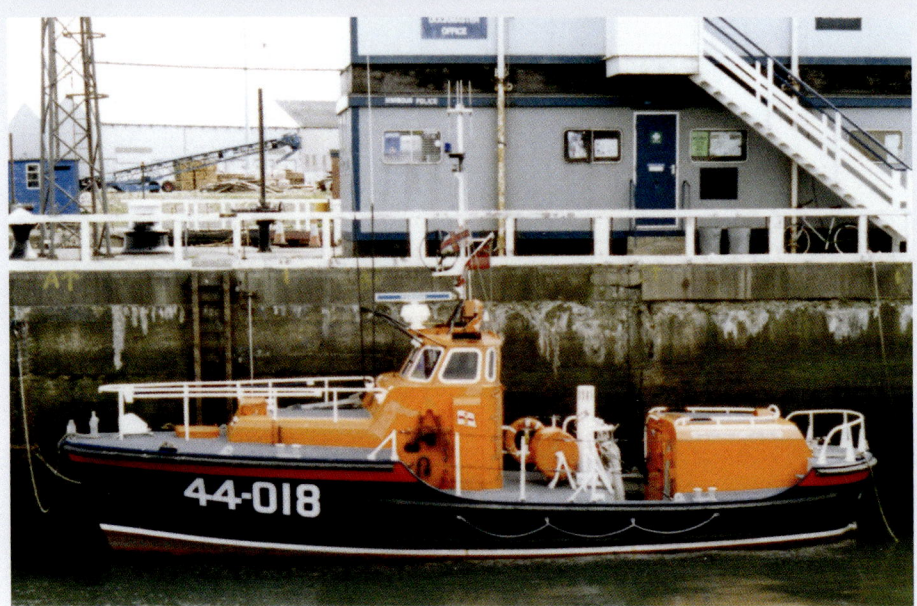

▲ 44-018 berthed at Hartlepool, the station she served for twenty years, 1994. (Nicholas Leach)

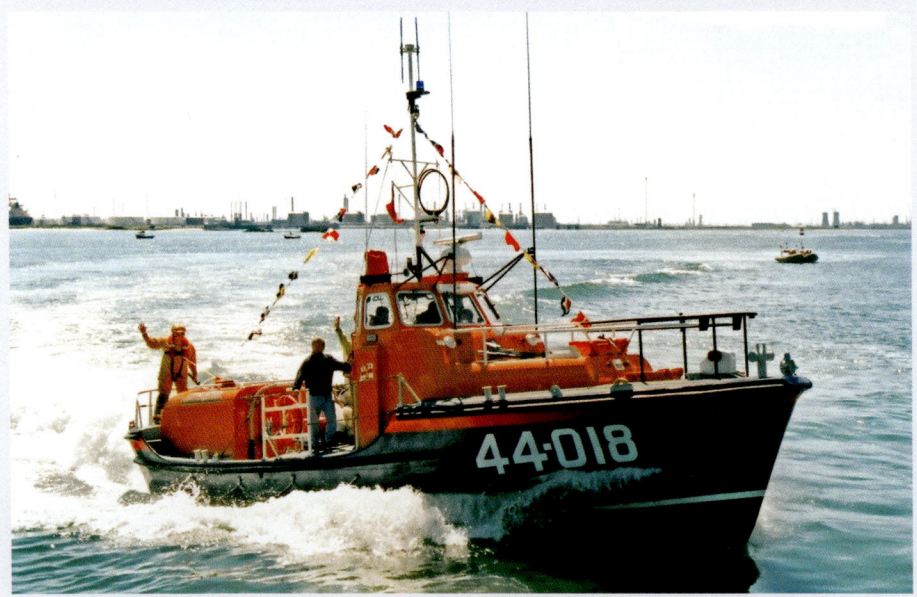

▲ 44-018 attending Teesmouth Lifeboat Day, July 1996. (Nicholas Leach)

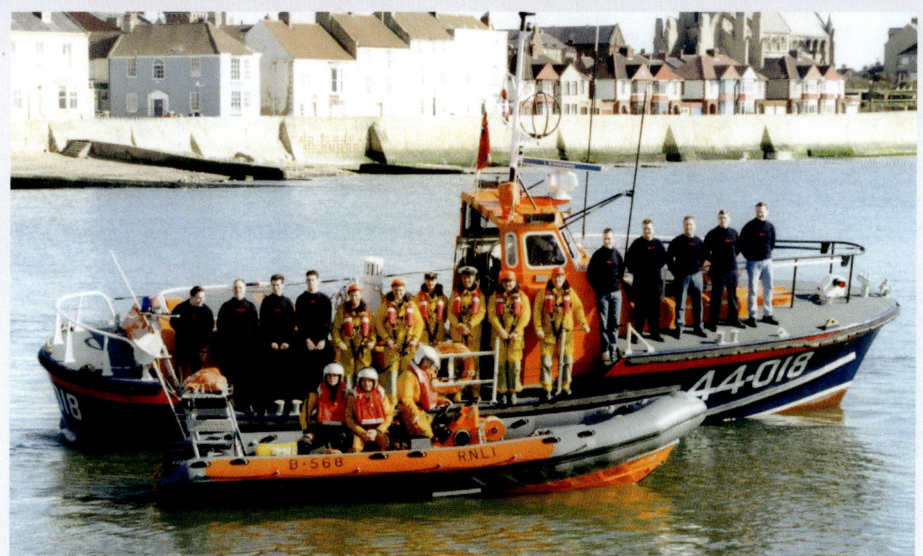

▲ 44-018 at Hartlepool with her crew and Atlantic 21 Burton Brewer (B-568).

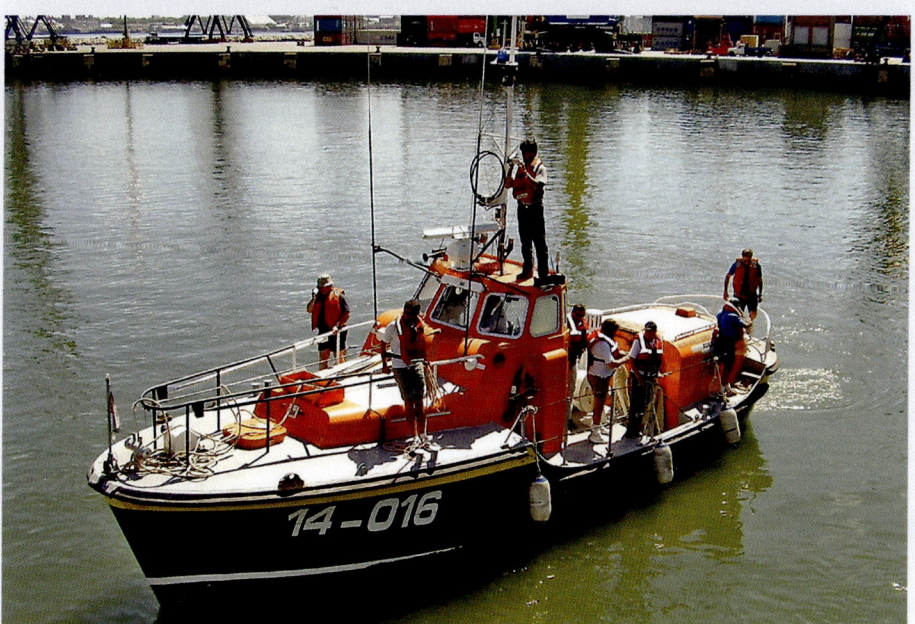

▲ 44-018 in service with ADES, the Uruguayian lifeboat service. She was stationed at Puerto del Buceo from 1997 to 2015. (By courtesy of Jorge Diena/ADES)

Louis Marchesi of Round Table

Key data

Built 1977, Bideford Shipyard, North Devon, yard no. Y62

Donor Gift of the National Association of Round Tables, Great Britain and Ireland

Named 18 Sep 1977 at Newhaven by Mrs Bangor-Jones, wife of the National President of
Round Tables, Great Britain and Ireland

Cost £139,823.50

Stations Newhaven 24 May 1977 – 9 Aug 1985 (289/134), Relief 9 Aug 1985 – Oct 1986 (0/0),
Alderney 23 Oct 1986 – 7 Mar 1994 (170/123), Exmouth 8 July 1994 – 6 July 1996 (39/5),
Relief 5 Dec 1996 – 20 Apr 1997 (1/0)

Disposal Sold 12.2.1999 to Waiheke Volunteer Coastguard, New Zealand

Service career

Louis Marchesi of Round Table had a varied RNLI career, serving at Newhaven for twelve years
before shorter stints at Alderney and Exmouth, completing a total of almost 500 services.
She faced extremely challenging conditions on 21 January 1980 when she was launched to the
cargo vessel Athina B, of Greece, which was in difficulties off Brighton Marina. The Shoreham
Harbour lifeboat succeeded in rescuing the vessel's crew of twenty-six, for which Coxswain Ken
Voice was awarded the Silver medal. Louis Marchesi of Round Table, under the command
of Coxswain/Mechanic Len Patten, faced exceptionally violent seas in severe force nine gale
winds, and was twice struck by enormous waves, the second of which caused a knockdown.
She was laid over on her beam ends, the wheelhouse was flooded and the capsize switches
activated, but the lifeboat righted herself, the engines were engaged and she continued. After
covering a further three miles in mountainous seas, a message was received that everyone on
board Athina B had been rescued so the lifeboat headed back for Newhaven. Although no
service had been performed on this occasion, the Waveney design had been tested to the limit.

After service

Louis Marchesi of Round Table was placed on the sale list on 29 May 1997 and sold out of
service on 12 February 1999 to the Royal New Zealand Coastguard. She left Tilbury in late February
1999, arrived in New Zealand in April, and was subsequently renamed P&O Nedlloyd Rescue, being
used as a rescue boat at Waiheke Island, off Auckland, by Waiheke Volunteer Coastguard.
In May 2006 she was sold by the Coastguard and became a privately-owned liveaboard
cruiser. In September 2010 she changed hands again and was kept on a swinging mooring in
Waitemata Harbour, Auckland, on the North Shore side just east of the Auckland Bridge.

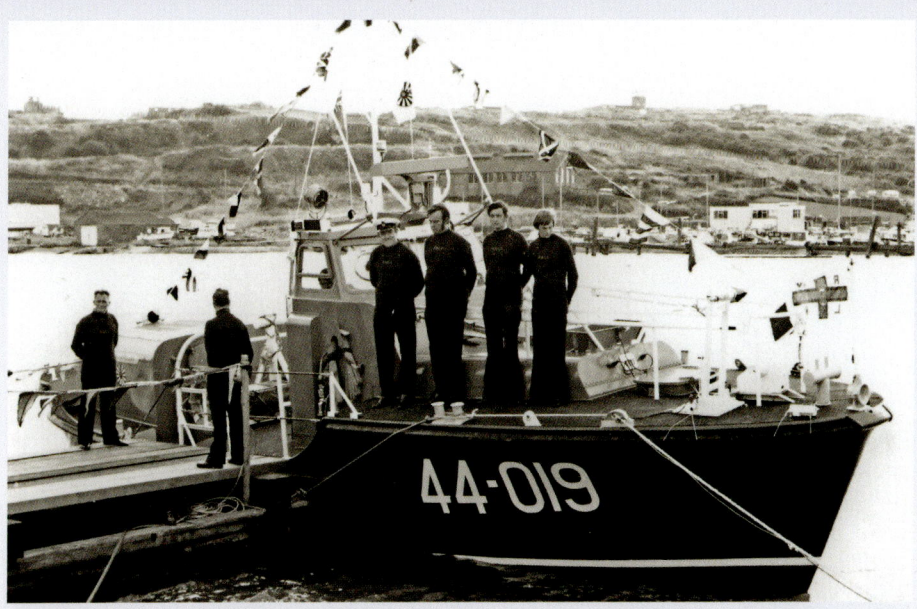

▲ 44-019 during her naming ceremony at Newhaven, 18 September 1977. (Jeff Morris)

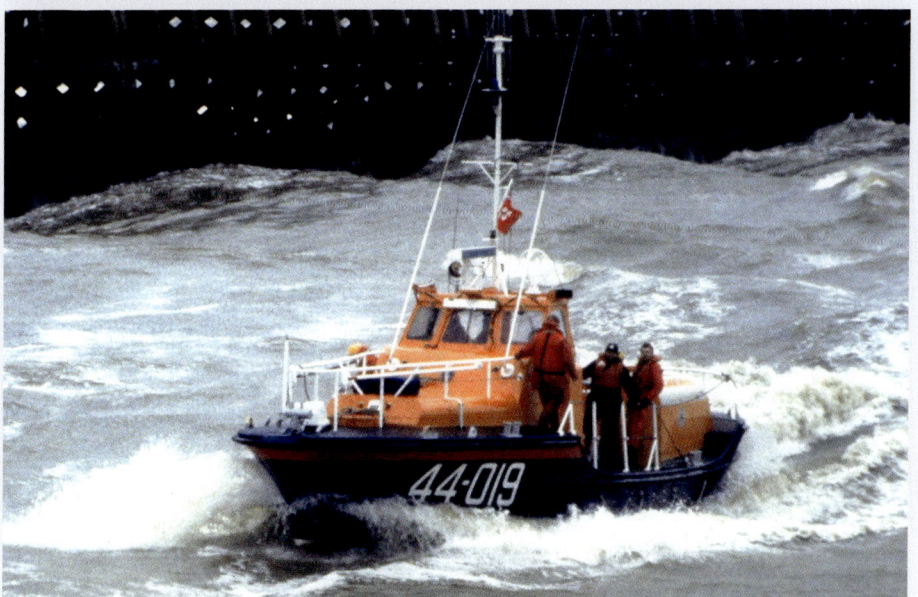

▲ 44-019 entering Newhaven harbour. (By courtesy of the RNLI)

Louis Marchesi of Round Table

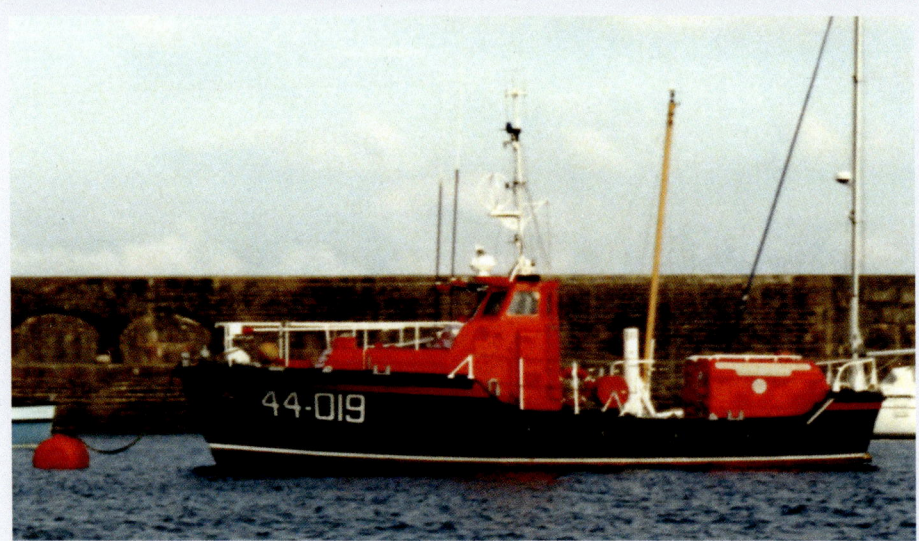

▲ 44-019 moored in Braye Harbour, Alderney, where she served for almost eight years.

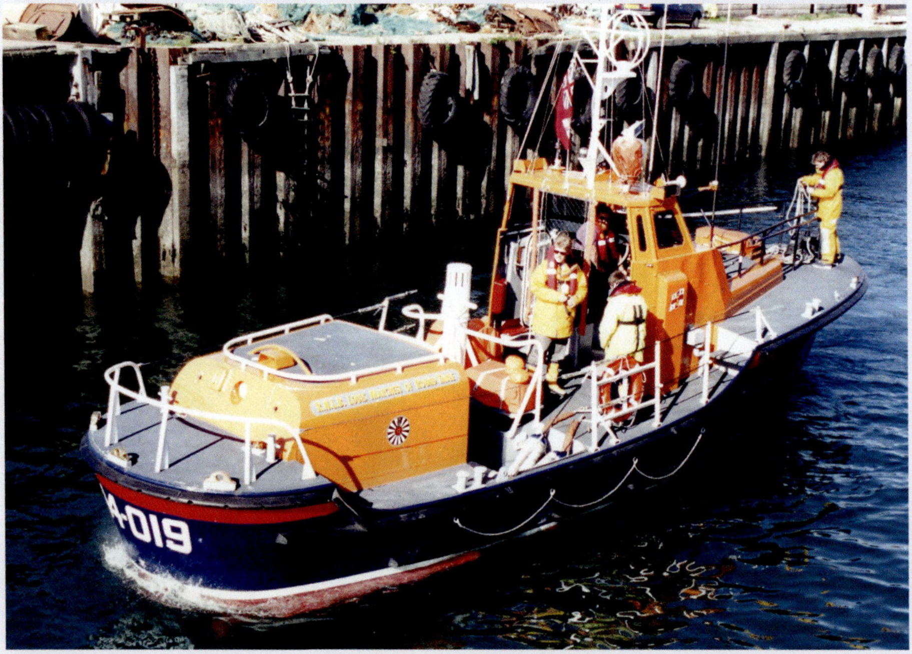

▲ 44-019 leaving Exmouth Dock on exercise, October 1994. (Nicholas Leach)

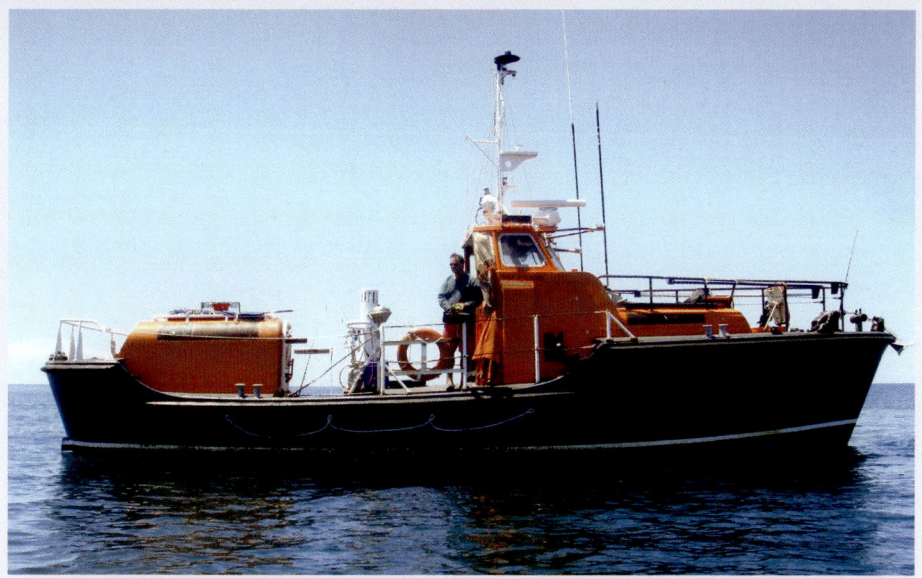

▲ 44-019 north of Port Jackson Bay on the Coromandel Peninsula, New Zealand, January 2012. (Armin Ziegler)

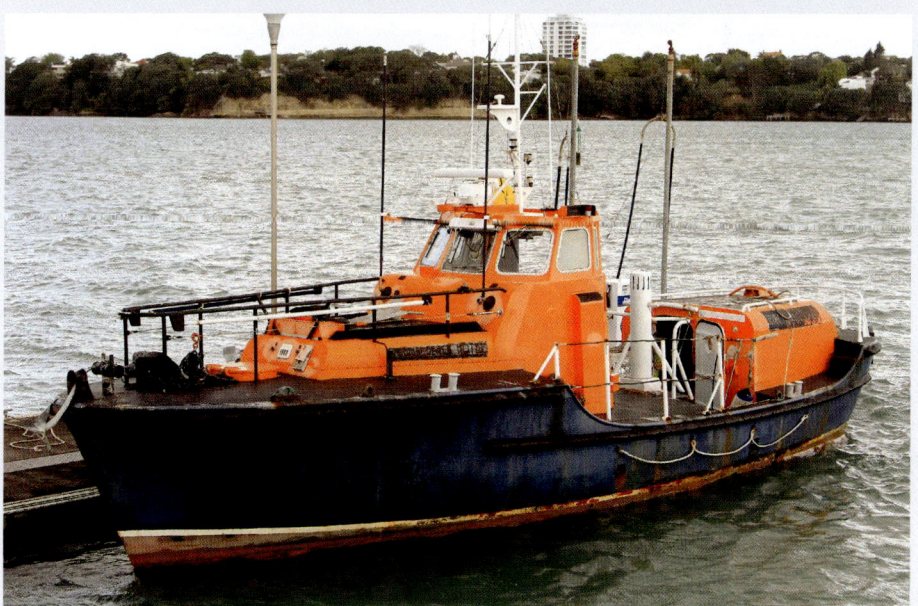

▲ 44-019 at Northcote Wharf, Northcote Point on Auckland's North Shore, October 2013. (Vic Young)

John Fison

Key data

Built 1980, Fairey Marine, Cowes, yard no. FM687
Donor Gifts of Mrs D. E. Fison, in memory of her husband; the John Jarrold Trust; and Mrs
D. Knowles; legacy of Mrs Annie Sutcliffe; and a gift from Fisons Ltd
Named 26 July 1980 at the Trinity House Pier, Harwich, by Mrs Dorothy E. Fison
Cost £243,487.34
Stations Harwich 11 Mar 1980 – 6 Oct 1996 (232/97), Relief 6 Oct 1996 – 24 Aug 1999 (25/3)
Disposal Sold 24 Aug 1999 to Raglan Volunteer Coastguard, New Zealand

Service career

John Fison was the second Waveney to serve at Harwich, and she spent more than sixteen years at the Essex station. She undertook a notable rescue on 19 December 1982 after the ferries European Gateway and Speedlink Vanguard were in collision off Felixstowe in winds gusting to force eight. Under the command of Coxswain/Mechanic Peter Burwood, John Fison picked up two unconscious men from the water, assisted one of the pilot vessels to recover a man from the water, and landed three bodies. Framed Letters of Thanks, signed by the RNLI Chairman, the Duke of Atholl, were presented to Coxswain/Mechanic Burwood and the Harwich crew. After her time at Harwich, John Fison briefly served as a relief lifeboat, with stints at Sheerness and Lowestoft. She spent more than a year at the Suffolk station, before going to the RNLI Depot, Poole, where she was stored before being sold out of service.

After service

John Fison was sold out of RNLI service on 24 August 1999 to the Royal New Zealand Coastguard. She left Tilbury Docks on 5 September 1999 and was transported on board the container ship New Zealand Pacific to Wellington, New Zealand, where she was unloaded on 22 October 1999. The engines were started, firing first time, and she then steamed to Mana, six hours around the coast, where she was lifted out of the water, cleaned and anti-fouled. After being put back into the water she was taken to Raglan, via New Plymouth, renamed Hamilton Rotary Rescue, and operated by the Volunteer Coastguard, being kept moored just off Raglan Wharf. Funding came from New Zealand National 'Loto' grants board, grant applications to local bodies and trusts, and the Royal New Zealand Coastguard Federation. In December 2005 she was sold by the Raglan Coastguard into private ownership at Napier. In 2007 she was sold again, being acquired by Harbour Services Australia, renamed Harbour Cruiser and used as a crew transfer and utility vessel at Fremantle.

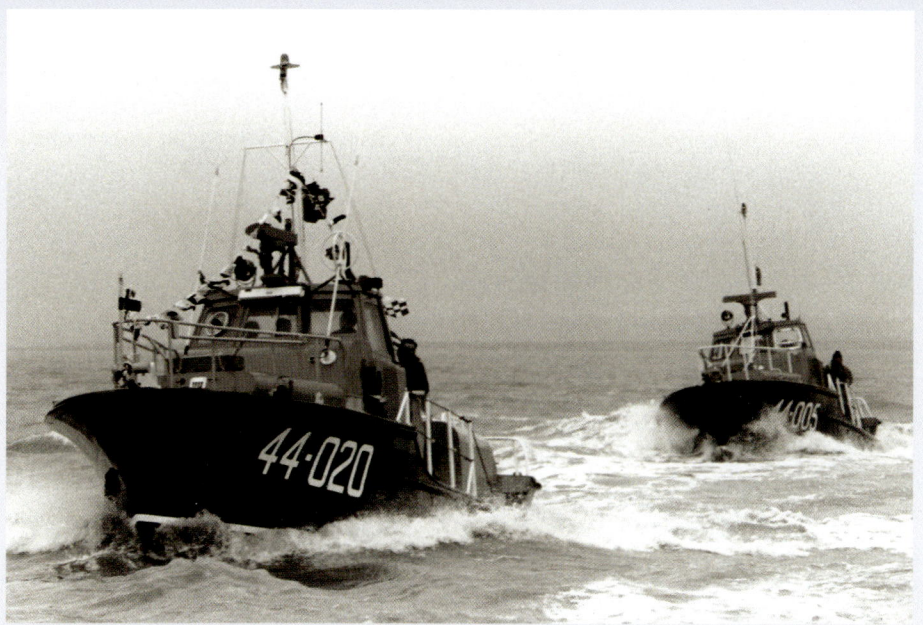

▲ 44-020 leading 44-005 into Harwich on the day she arrived on station, 10 March 1980. (Harwich RNLI)

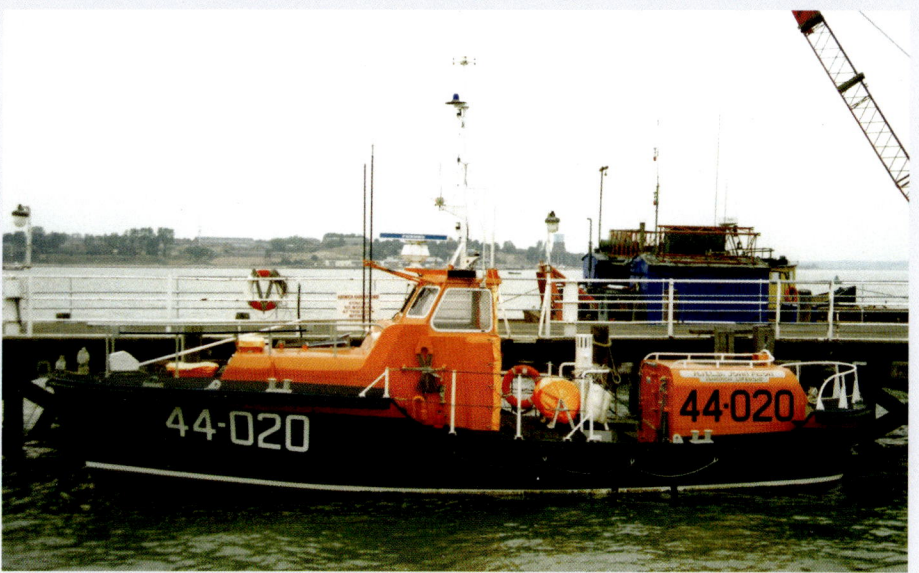

▲ 44-020 on station at Harwich, at moorings in the Pound, August 1989. (Nicholas Leach)

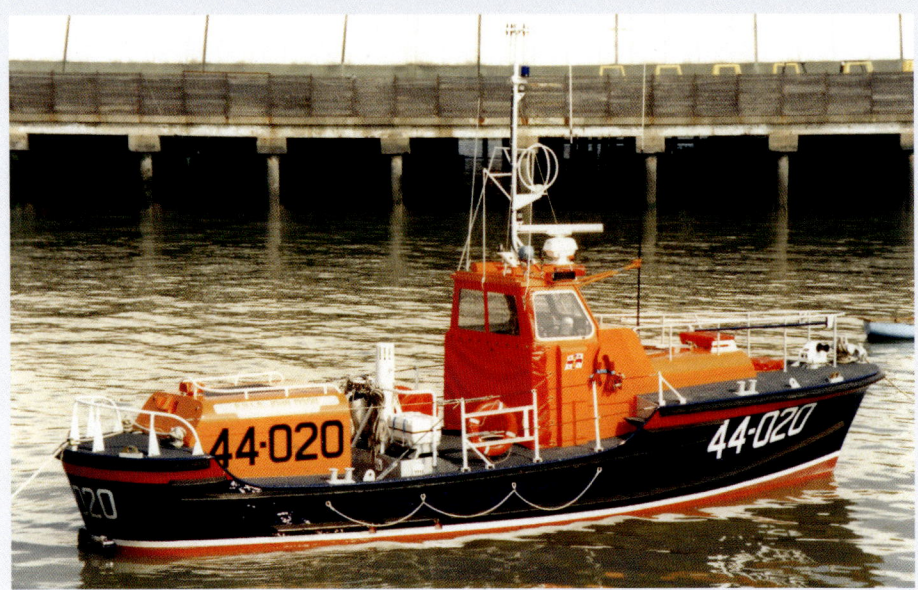

▲ 44-020 moored at Navyard Wharf, Harwich, May 1995. (Nicholas Leach)

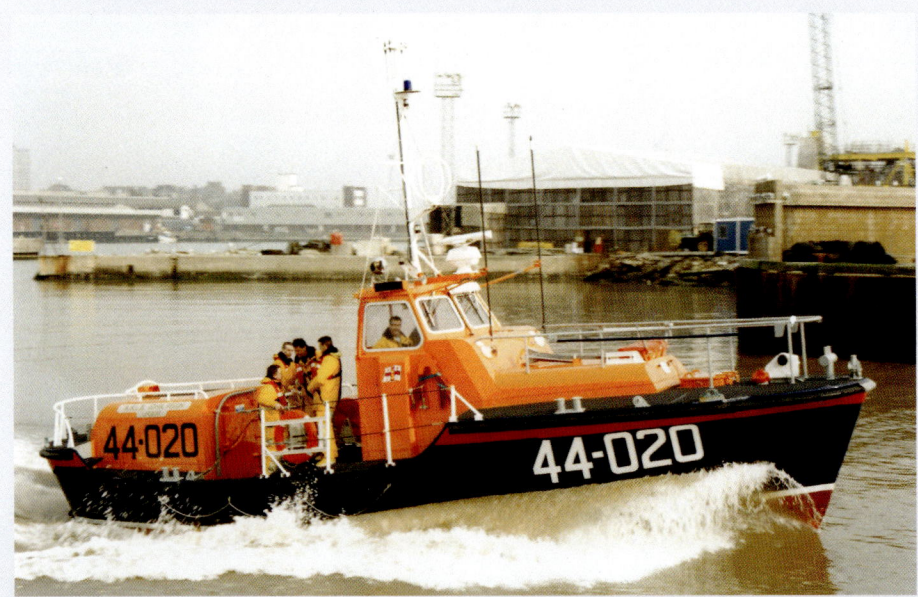

▲ 44-020 leaving on exercise while on relief duty at Lowestoft, March 1998. She served at Lowestoft from October 1997 to November 1998, launching twenty-five times on service and saving three lives. (Nicholas Leach)

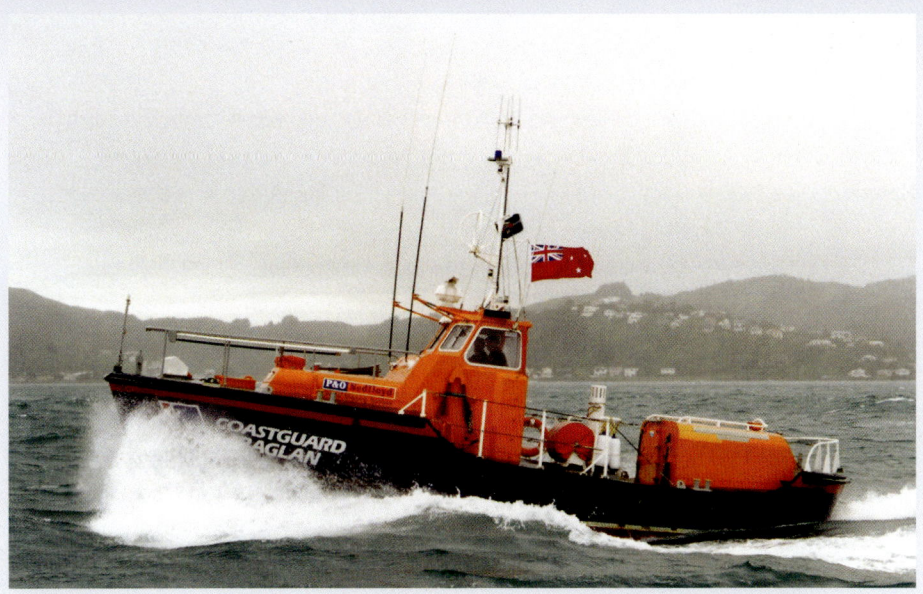

▲ 44-020 was renamed Hamilton Rotary Rescue for service with Raglan Coastguard. (V.H. Young)

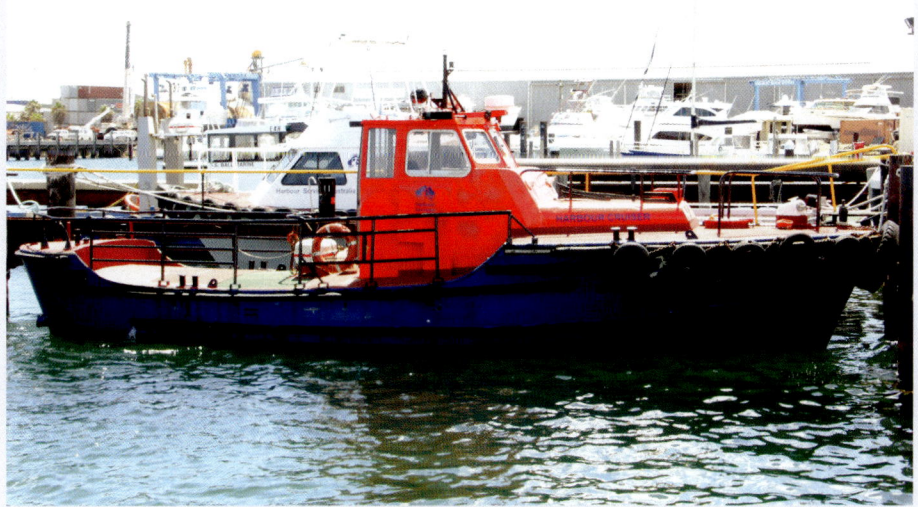

▲ 44-020 renamed Harbour Cruiser and used as a crew transfer and utility vessel at Fremantle, having had her aft cabin removed and her wheelhouse partially enclosed.

Barham

Key data

Built 1980, Fairey Marine, Cowes, yard no. FM694

Donor Legacies of Mr Colin A.S. Stringer, Walton-on-Thames, and Mrs A. Geraldine Miles, Southbourne, West Sussex. The Barham Survivors' Association funded equipment

Named 17 Sep 1980 at Gorleston-on-Sea by Mrs Angela Guillaume, to commemorate those who lost their lives in HMS Barham in 1941

Stations Gorleston 30 May 1980 – Mar 1996 (254/71), Relief Apr 1996 – 1999 (25/11)

Disposal Sold Nov 1999 to Royal New Zealand Volunteer Coastguard

Service career

Barham served at Great Yarmouth & Gorleston in Norfolk for almost sixteen years, with a further three years in the Relief Fleet. During her time at Gorleston, Barham undertook a number of outstanding rescues, including one on 3 May 1982, when she saved the yacht Seamist of Rhu, which was aground on the Scroby Sands, and rescued the yacht's two crew in a north-easterly gale and rough seas. Lifeboat crew member Paul Carter had to be transferred to the yacht to assist with rigging a towline in order to pull the yacht clear. In recognition of his skill and determination, Coxswain/Mechanic Richard Hawkins was accorded the Thanks Inscribed on Vellum for this service. Another fine rescue was performed on the night of 18-19 November 1986, when Barham rescued two crew from the rig support vessel Seaforth Conqueror, which was aground on the North Scroby Sands in a south-westerly storm and very rough seas. The Caister Volunteer Lifeboat Shirley Jean Adye also went out, under the command of Coxswain Roland Read, and rescued ten of the vessel's crew. The Thanks Inscribed on Vellum were accorded to both Coxswain/Mechanic Hawkins and also to Coxswain Read.

After service

Barham was placed on the sale list on 18 January 1999 and sold out of service in 1999 to the Royal New Zealand Coastguard, who operated her as a lifeboat at Napier, Hawke's Bay, renamed Legend. In June 2003, deemed unsuitable for Coastguard operations, she was sold for about NZ$80,000 (£25,000) to Graham Booth and Fiona Rolfe, who converted her in Auckland into a more practical boat. They removed the aft cabin, extended and enclosed the wheelhouse and installed six berths. They also fitted a dinghy cradle, a new winch and a plough anchor. She was used as a pleasure boat and for dive charter work. In 2008 she was bought by Wayne Fisk, who kept her at Seaview Marina, Wellington. In 2012 she was offered for sale from Auckland Shipbrokers Limited for NZD $170,000.

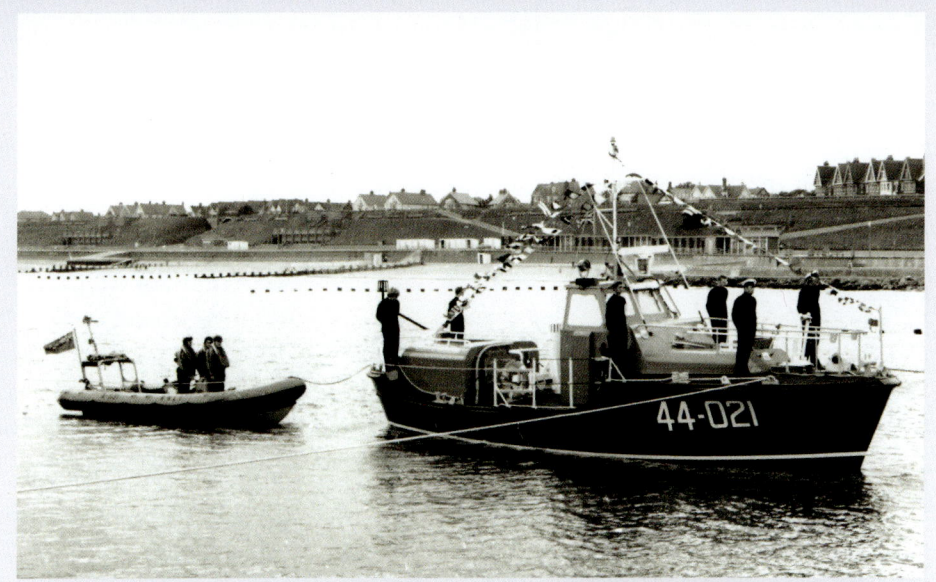

▲ 44-021 during her naming ceremony at Gorleston, 17 September 1980. (Jeff Morris)

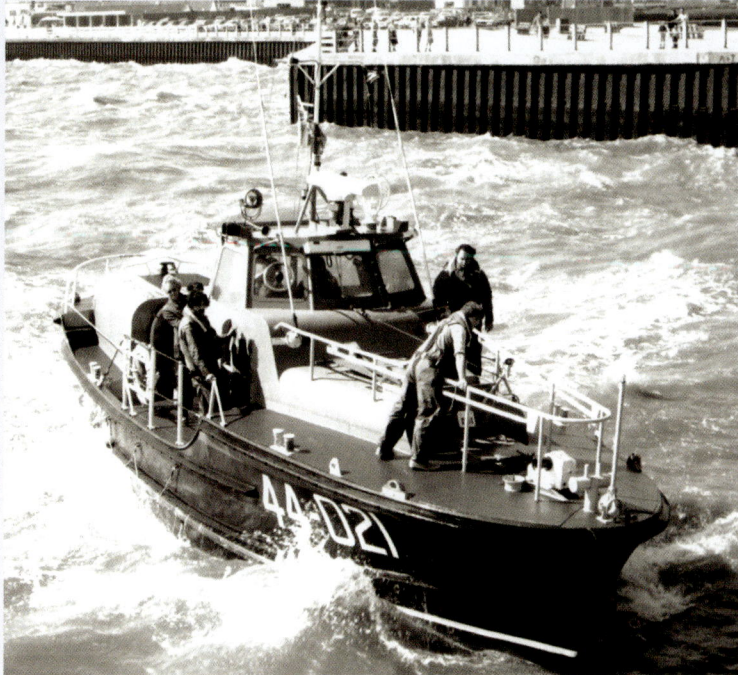

◄ 44-021 on exercise off the entrance to Gorleston Harbour. (J.W. Markham)

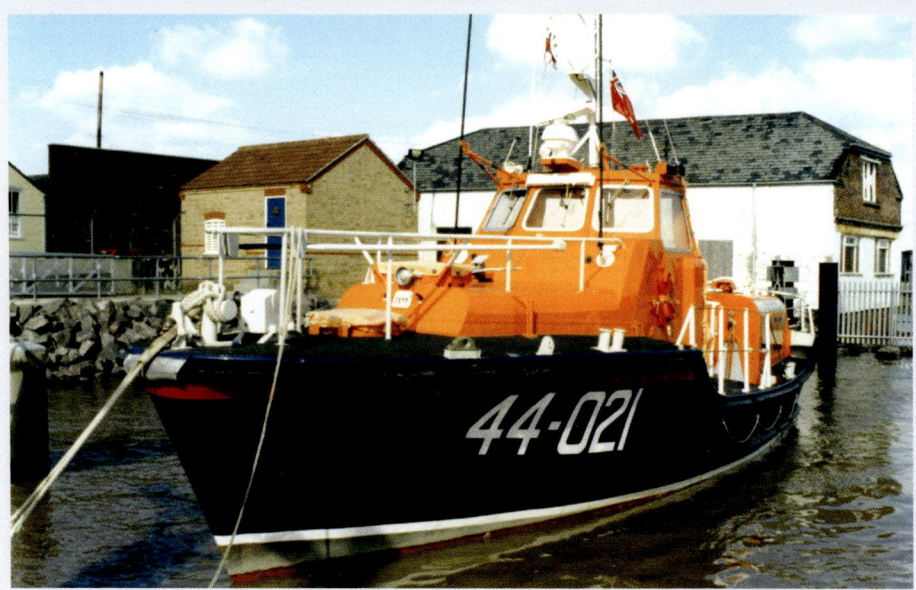

▲ 44-021 in the mooring pen at Gorleston, March 1995. (Nicholas Leach)

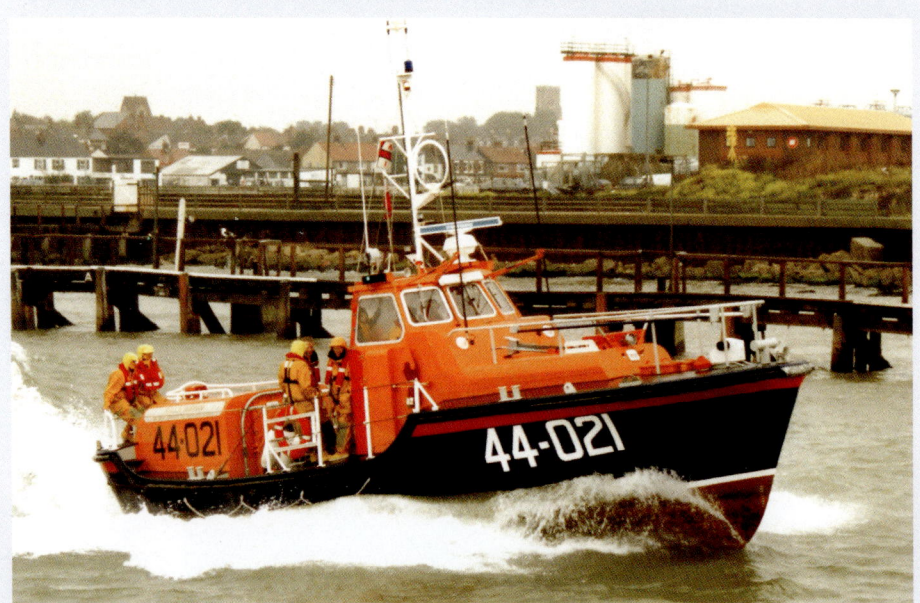

▲ 44-021 leaving Gorleston on exercise, September 1995. (Nicholas Leach)

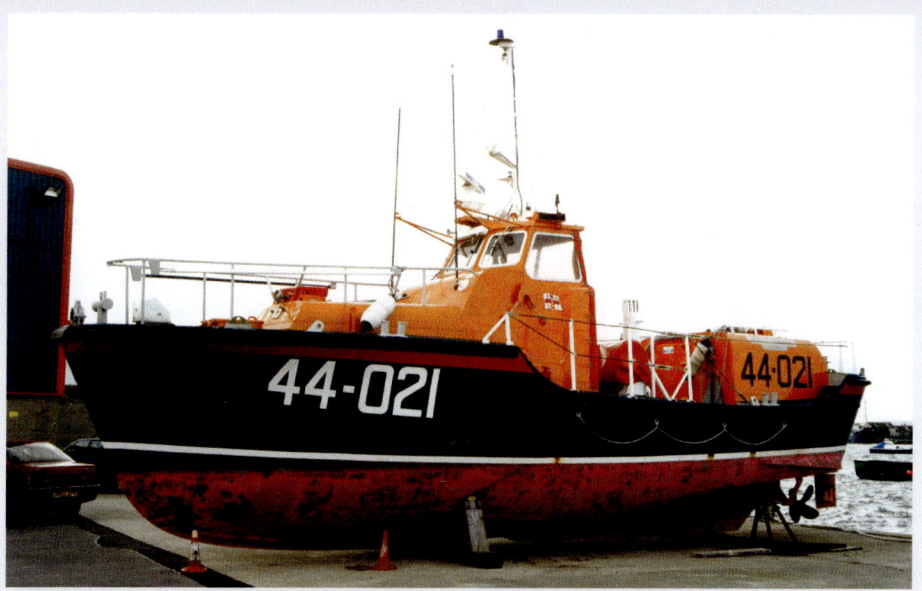

▲ 44-021 at the RNLI Depot, Poole, awaiting sale, February 1999. (Nicholas Leach)

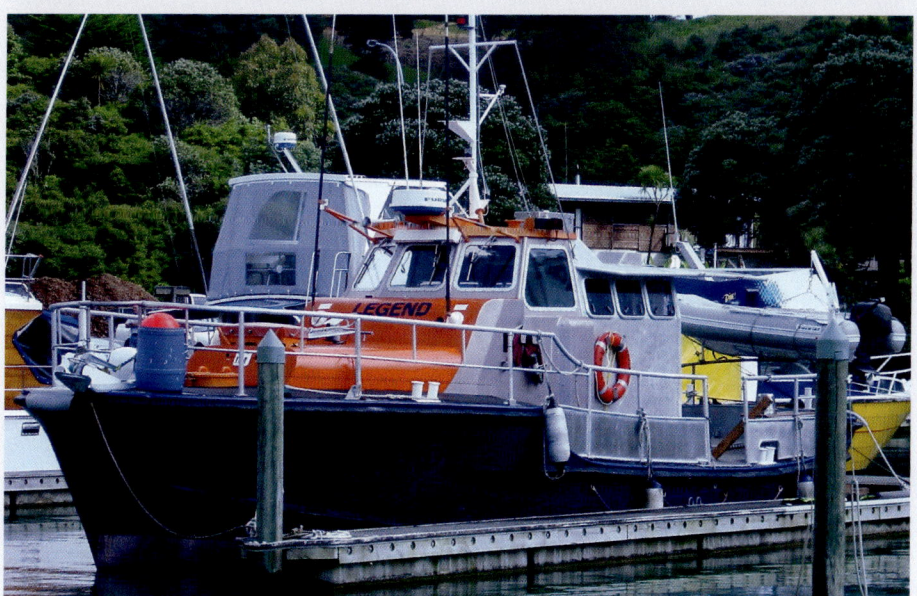

▲ 44-021 renamed Legend at Seaview Marina, Wellington, November 2004. (Graham Booth)

The William and Jane

Key data

Built 1982, Fairey Allday Marine, Cowes, yard no. FM710

Donor Legacies of Miss Mabel Hewson, Mrs Mary Grey, Mrs Rhoda Whittaker, Mr L.G.A. Dunn and Frank Rowe

Named 17 Sep 1983 at Dun Cow Quay, Blyth, by Her Grace the Duchess of Northumberland, after the parents of donor Miss Hewson

Stations Blyth 26 Oct 1982 – Dec 1995 (136/43); Larne 19 Mar 1996 – Nov 1998 (23/11)

Disposal Sold out of service May 1999 to the Royal New Zealand Coastguard Federation

Service career

The William and Jane was the last Waveney to be built. She served at Blyth for just over thirteen years, followed by a further two and a half years at Larne, in Northern Ireland, where she was the first all-weather lifeboat at the new station on the Antrim coast, established to improve rescue coverage in the Irish Sea. The most notable rescue in which she was involved was undertaken on 7 December 1982 while she was serving at Blyth, when she was launched to the fishing vessel Castle Cove, which was taking water five miles off the Tyne. In force seven winds, the lifeboat encountered heavy breaking seas as she left harbour. Once on scene, the lifeboat crew rigged a tow and, in breaking seas up to 20ft high, headed for the Tyne at quarter speed. The five-mile tow took over an hour, but, as the two craft approached the Tyne, the fishing vessel began to sink. The tow line was slipped and the lifeboat came alongside the vessel, which had heeled over, and the three fishermen were pulled aboard. For this rescue, Coxswain Hatcher was awarded the Bronze medal and Medal Service Certificates were presented to the rest of the crew.

After service

The William and Jane was sold out of service in May 1999 to the Royal New Zealand Coastguard Federation, being renamed John Barton Acland Rescue. She was stationed at Kaikoura until 27 June 2004, when she was taken to Picton and put up for sale. In May 2005 she was bought by Tom and Kris Carpenter, of Hawaii, and renamed Gryphon. She stayed at Picton initially but has subsequently travelled extensively, after being converted internally, though remaining little altered externally from her service days. She was based at Opua, Bay of Islands, New Zealand from April 2012 to July 2016, when she was taken to Newport, near Sydney, Australia. In February 2018 she was taken to California, going from Australia to Ensenada, Mexico on board the yacht transfer ship Yacht Express, and was then sailed up the California coast to a new base, with a new pontoon for her use and a boathouse nearby.

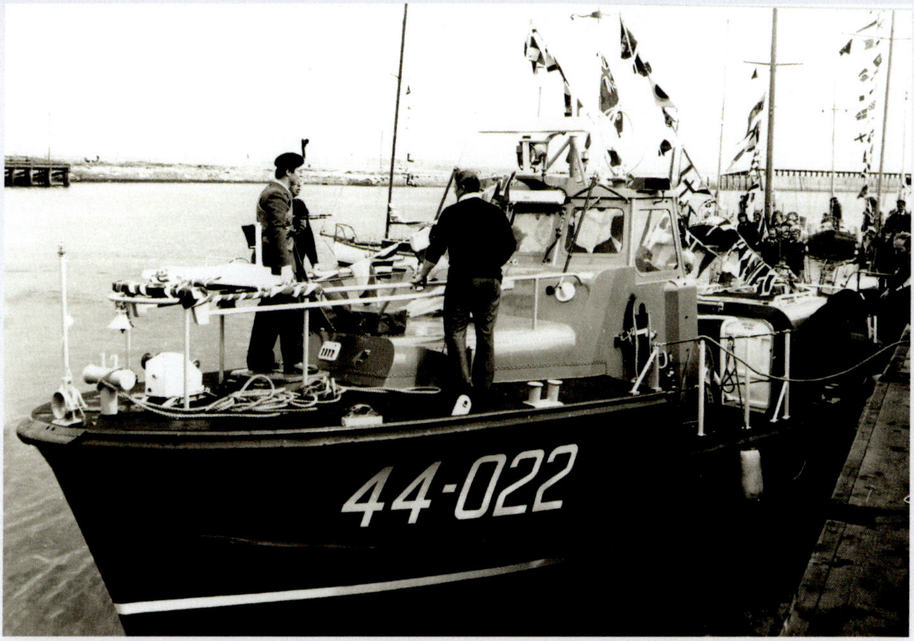

▲ 44-022 at Dun Cow Quay, Blyth, for her naming ceremony on 17 September 1983. (Jeff Morris)

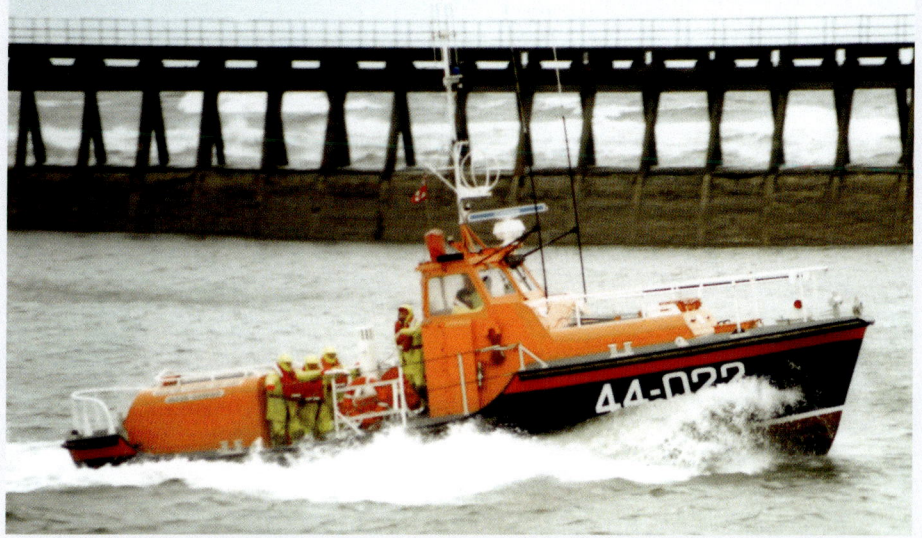

▲ 44-022 heading out of Blyth Harbour on exercise, September 1991. (Brian Chandler)

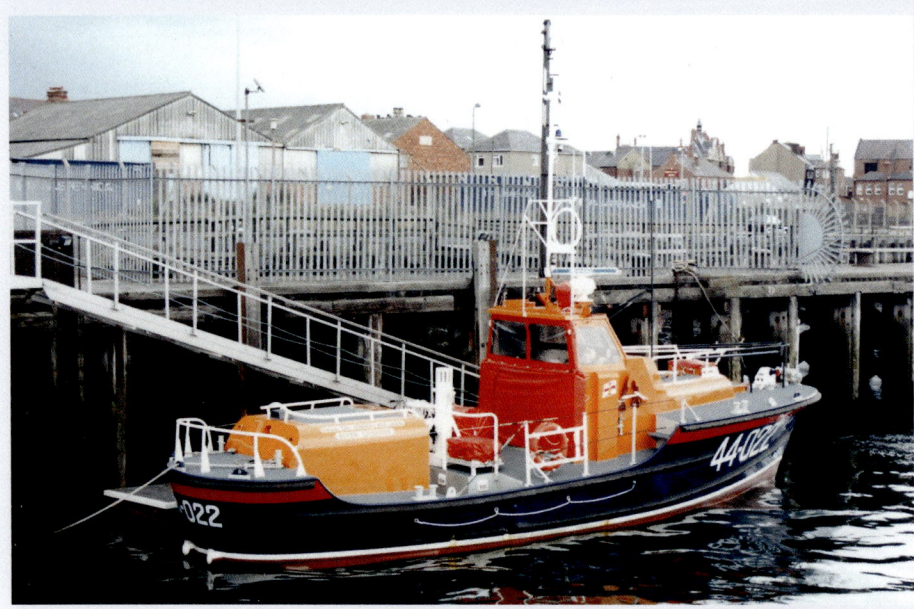

▲ 44-021 on station at Blyth, August 1994. (Nicholas Leach)

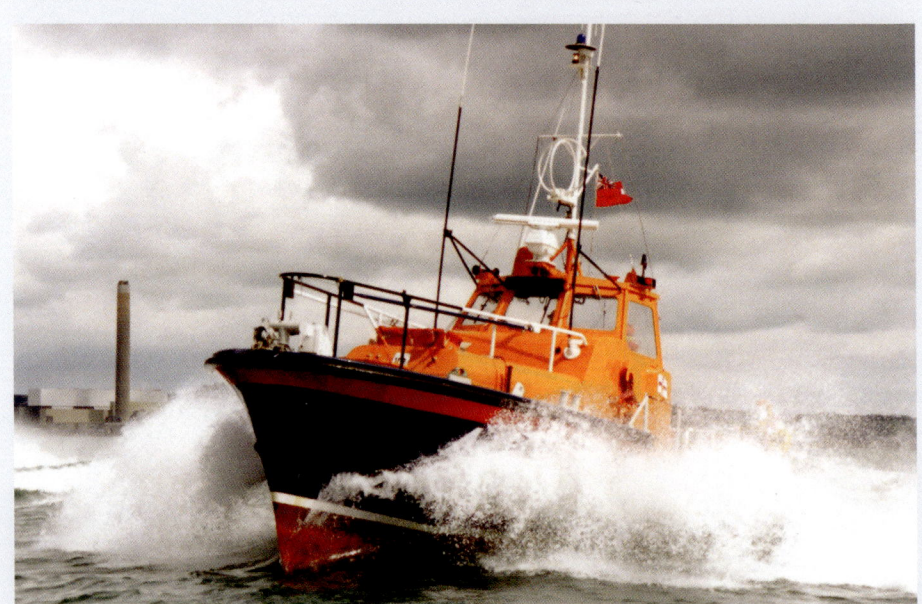

▲ 44-021 at Larne just before leaving service, 1998; she was the last Waveney in Ireland. (By courtesy of RNLI)

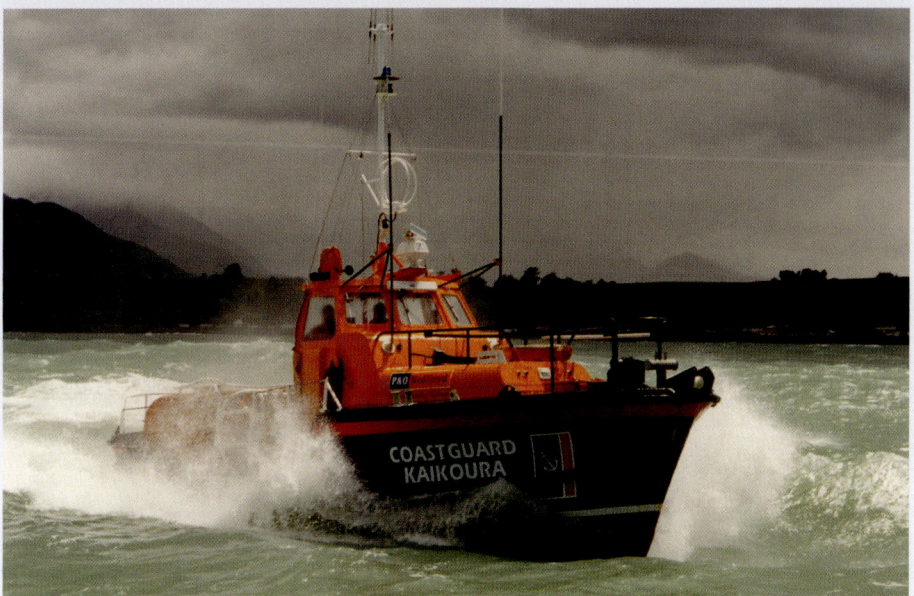

▲ 44-022 was stationed at Kaikoura on South Island, NZ, renamed John Barton Acland Rescue. (V.H. Young)

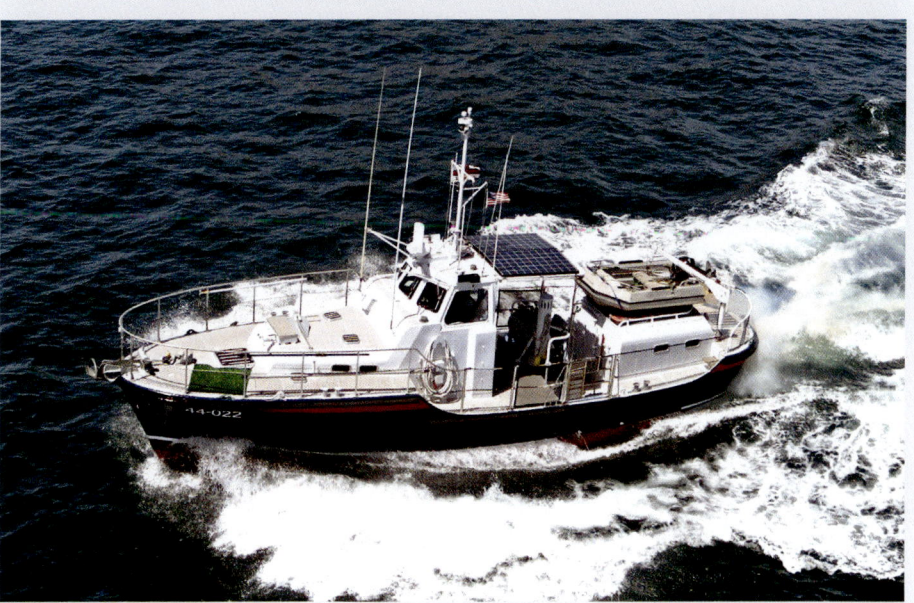

▲ 44-022 was sold into private ownership and renamed Gryphon to be used for coastal cruising.

MEDAL-WINNING SERVICES

Year	Date	Lifeboat (Op No)	Station	Casualty	Medal	Recipients
1969	9 Nov	Khami (44-003)	Gorleston	Motor vessel Karen Bravo	Bronze	Coxswain John Bryan
1974	13 Dec	Khami (44-003)	Gorleston	Motor vessel Biscaya	Bronze	Coxswain John Bryan
1975	16 Aug	Helen Turnbull (44-009)	Sheerness	Yacht Eladnit	Bronze	Coxswain Charles Bowry
1975	1 Dec	Faithful Forester (44-004)	Dover	Coaster Primrose	Silver Bronze	Coxswain Arthur Liddon Second Coxswain Anthony Hawkins
1976	9 Jul	St Patrick (44-014)	Dunmore East	Small motor boat	Bronze	Coxswain/Mechanic Stephen Whittle
1978	15 Feb	Thomas Forehead and Mary Rowse II (44-010)	Plymouth	Trawler Elly Gerda	Bronze Bronze	Acting Coxswain Patrick Marshall Mechanic Cyril Alcock
1978	30 Dec	Helen Turnbull (44-009)	Sheerness	Cabin cruiser Ma Jolie II	Bronze	Coxswain Charles Bowry
1979	22 Dec	Khami (44-003)	Gorleston	Fishing vessel St Margarite	Bronze	Coxswain Richard Hawkins
1980	19 Mar	Helen Turnbull (44-009)	Sheerness	Radio ship Mi Amigo	Silver	Coxswain Charles Bowry
1980	12 Sep	Connel Elizabeth Cargill (44-007)	Troon	Dredger Holland I	Silver	Coxswain Ian Johnson
1982	7 Dec	The William and Jane (44-022)	Blyth	Fishing vessel Castle Cove	Bronze	Coxswain Charles Hatcher
1982	14 Dec	Faithful Forester (44-004)	St Helier (relief)	Yacht Festina Lente III	Bronze	Coxswain Michael Berry
1983	3 Sep	Thomas James King (44-013)	St Helier	Yacht Cythara	Silver	Coxswain Michael Berry
1985	10 Nov	The Scout (44-018)	Hartlepool	Motor vessel Anne	Bronze	Coxswain Robbie Maiden
1985	26 Dec	Ralph and Joy Swann (44-016)	Ramsgate	Trawler Gloire à Marie II	Silver	Coxswain Ron Cannon
1987	16 Oct	Helen Turnbull (44-009)	Sheerness	Cabin cruiser	Bronze	Coxswain Robin Castle
1988	9 Apr	The White Rose of Yorkshire (44-012)	Whitby	Yacht Cymba	Bronze	Coxswain Peter Thomson
1990	6 Oct	44-001	Eyemouth (relief)	Missing divers	Silver	Acting Coxswain James Dougal

AFTER SERVICE SUMMARY

Op No	ON	Station(s)	Replacement	Sold	Renamed	Current location
44-001		Relief	—	—	44-001	Chatham Dockyard
44-002	1001	Dun Laoghaire	Waveney 44-015	1996	Sarah JFK/ Fortitude	Lagos, Nigeria
44-003	1002	Gorleston	Waveney 44-021	1999	P&O Nedlloyd Stratheden/ Khami	Beauty Point, Launceston, Tasmania
44-004	1003	Dover Holyhead	50ft Thames 47ft Tyne	1999	P&O Nedlloyd Strathmore/ Harbour Conquest	Fremantle, Australia
44-005	1004	Harwich Amble	Waveney 44-020 12m Mersey	1999	St Hilda of Whitby	Whitby, North Yorkshire
44-006	1005	Barry Dock Donaghadee Courtmacsherry	52ft Arun 52ft Arun 14m Trent	1999	P&O Nedlloyd Strathallan/ Harbour Crusader	Fremantle, Australia, scrapped 2019
44-007	1006	Troon Arklow	Waveney 44-011 Waveney 44-011	1999	P&O Nedlloyd Rawalpindi	Brisbane River, Queensland, Australia
44-008	1026	Eyemouth	14m Trent	1999	The Spirit of Standard Bank	Lüderitz, Namibia
44-009	1027	Sheerness Achill Island	14m Trent 52ft Arun	1998	Badger/ Sturm	Bowling Canal Basin, West Dunbartonshire
44-010	1028	Plymouth Fowey	52ft Arun 14m Trent	1999	Westgate Rescue/ Harrier	Fiordland, South Island, New Zealand
44-011	1029	Poole Troon Arklow	33ft Brede 52ft Arun 14m Trent	1999	P&O Nedlloyd Strathaird/ Augustine Courtauld	Melbourne, Australia
44-012	1033	Whitby Invergordon	47ft Tyne 14m Trent	1999	IA.001/ The White Rose of Yorkshire	Canoe Pass, Ladner, BC Canada
44-013	1034	St Helier Dunbar	47ft Tyne 14m Trent	1998	North Esk/ Ledra Express	Limassol, Cyprus
44-014	1035	Dunmore East	14m Trent	1999	P&O Nedlloyd Strathnaver/ Community Spirit/ St Patrick Strathnaver	Western Port, Victoria, Australia
44-015	1036	Fleetwood Dun Laoghaire	47ft Tyne 14m Trent	1996	St Boisil	Berwick-upon-Tweed
44-016	1042	Ramsgate Tobermory Portree	47ft Tyne 54ft Arun 14m Trent	1998	West Swann	Port Howard, West Falkland
44-017	1043	Donaghadee Sunderland	Waveney 44-006 14m Trent	1997	Nicholsons Rescue/ Trust Porirua Rescue/ Toucan	Whanganui River, New Zealand
44-018	1044	Hartlepool	47ft Tyne	1997	ADES 16/Montemar S.A.	Montevideo, Uruguay
44-019	1045	Newhaven Alderney Exmouth	52ft Arun 14m Trent 14m Trent	1999	P&O Nedlloyd Rescue/ Louis Marchesi of Round Table	Auckland, New Zealand
44-020	1060	Harwich	17m Severn	1999	Hamilton Rotary Rescue/ Harbour Cruiser	Fremantle, Australia
44-021	1065	Gorleston	14m Trent	1999	Waveney/ Legend	Wellington, N Zealand
44-022	1079	Blyth Larne	14m Trent 52ft Arun	1999	John Barton Acland Rescue/ Gryphon	Newport, Oregon, USA

WAVENEY LIFEBOATS

Stations served by the Waveney lifeboats

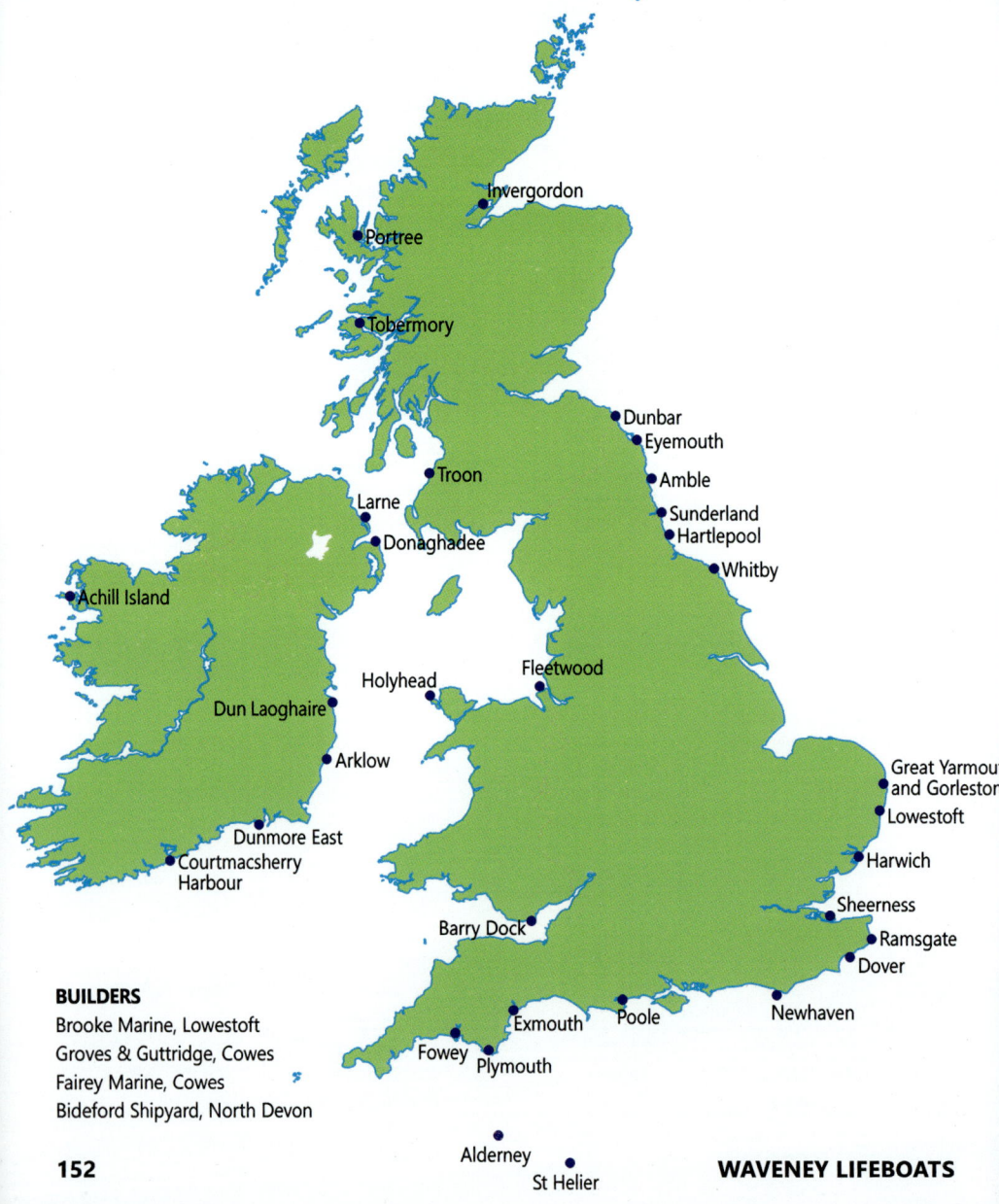

- Invergordon
- Portree
- Tobermory
- Dunbar
- Eyemouth
- Troon
- Amble
- Larne
- Sunderland
- Donaghadee
- Hartlepool
- Whitby
- Achill Island
- Fleetwood
- Holyhead
- Dun Laoghaire
- Arklow
- Great Yarmout and Gorleston
- Lowestoft
- Dunmore East
- Harwich
- Courtmacsherry Harbour
- Sheerness
- Barry Dock
- Ramsgate
- Dover
- Newhaven
- Exmouth
- Poole
- Fowey
- Plymouth
- Alderney
- St Helier

BUILDERS

Brooke Marine, Lowestoft
Groves & Guttridge, Cowes
Fairey Marine, Cowes
Bideford Shipyard, North Devon

WAVENEY LIFEBOATS